Prentice Hall Health

Q&A review

for Phlebotomy

Fifth Edition

Kathleen Becan-McBride, EdD, MT(ASCP)
Director, Community Outreach and Education
Coordinator, Texas-Mexico Border Health Services
Professor, UT-H Medical School, Dept. of Family Practice and
Community Medicine
School of Public Health, School of Nursing
The University of Texas-Houston Health Science Center
Texas Medical Center, Houston, Texas
Assistant Director for Academic Partnerships, Greater Houston AHEC

Diana Garza, EdD, MT(ASCP), CLS
Associate Research Professor
Office of Interdisciplinary Health Care Education
Texas Woman's University-Houston Center
Adjunct Associate Professor
Department of Laboratory Medicine
The University of Texas M.D. Anderson Cancer Center
Texas Medical Center, Houston, Texas

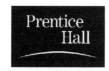

Prentice Hall
Upper Saddle River, New Jersey 07458

Library of Congress Cataloging-in-Publication Data
Becan-McBride, Kathleen, 1949–
    Prentice Hall health Q&A review for Phlebotomy,
    Fifth edition / Kathleen Becan-McBride, Diana Garza.
        p. ; cm.
    Includes bibliographical references and index.
    ISBN 0-13-088715-3 (alk. paper)
        1. Phlebotomy—Examinations, questions, etc. I. Garza, Diana
    II. Title.
        [DNLM: 1. Phlebotomy—Examination Questions.
        QY 39 G245p 1999 Suppl. 2001]
    RB45.15 .G37 1999 Suppl.
    616.07′561—dc21
                                                    00-059861

Publisher: Julie Alexander
Executive Editor: Greg Vis
Acquisitions Editors: Mark Cohen and Barbara Krawiec
Managing Development Editor: Marilyn Meserve
Director of Production and Manufacturing: Bruce Johnson
Managing Production Editor: Patrick Walsh
Production Editor: Carol Eckhart, York Production Services
Production Liaison: Danielle Newhouse
Manufacturing Manager: Ilene Sanford
Creative Director: Marianne Frasco
Cover Design Coordinator: Maria Guglielmo
Cover and Interior Designer: Janice Bielawa
Director of Marketing: Leslie Cavaliere
Marketing Coordinator: Cindy Frederick
Editorial Assistants: Melissa Kerian and Mary Ellen Ruitenberg
Composition: York Production Services
Printing and Binding: The Banta Company

Prentice-Hall International (UK) Limited, *London*
Prentice-Hall of Australia Pty. Limited, *Sydney*
Prentice-Hall Canada Inc., *Toronto*
Prentice-Hall Hispanoamericana, S.A., *Mexico*
Prentice-Hall of India Private Limited, *New Delhi*
Prentice-Hall of Japan, Inc., *Tokyo*
Prentice-Hall Singapore Pte. Ltd.
Editora Prentice-Hall do Brasil, Ltda., *Rio de Janeiro*

*To my husband, Mark;
my sons, Patrick and Jonathan;
my parents; my sister; and my parents-in-law
for their support and devotion.*

Kathleen Becan-McBride

*To my husband, Peter McLaughlin; my children,
Lauren, Kaitlin, and Kevin; and my parents
for their affection, patience, and constant support.*

Diana Garza

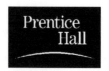

10 9 8 7 6 5 4 3 2 1
ISBN 0-13-088715-3

Prentice Hall Health

Q&A review

for Phlebotomy

Contents

SECTION V: Quality Management and Legal Issues 219

APPENDICES: Medical Measurement, Formulas, and Symbols 241

Preface

The number of clinical laboratory techniques, automated instruments, and analyses continues to escalate, increasing the demand for proper collection of patient laboratory specimens. Since the majority of laboratory errors occurs in the preanalytical phase, it is essential that health care students and practitioners who are responsible for blood and specimen collections (i.e., phlebotomists, clinical laboratory technologists and technicians, nurses, respiratory therapists, and others) have an in-depth knowledge of their professional responsibilities. National board certification in phlebotomy is required by many health care institutions, clinics, and physicians' offices as a result of federal, safety, and quality assurance requirements. In addition, the rationale for phlebotomy state licensure is gaining momentum across the nation. Because of these laws and to ensure high-quality patient care, continuing education in phlebotomy safety and quality assurance has become paramount.

These important events in the responsibilities of blood collection have served to shape the fifth edition of *Prentice Hall Health Q&A Review for Phlebotomy.* It has been designed to act as a study companion for those who are (1) preparing for national or state board certification/licensure examinations and/or (2) pursuing self-assessment in blood collection.

Prentice Hall Health Q&A Review for Phlebotomy, Fifth Edition, includes over 650 multiple-choice questions as a means to the overall review of blood collection, handling, and transportation. The chapters in this book are sequenced to match the order in *Phlebotomy Handbook: Blood Collection Essentials, Fifth Edition.* The questions and answer content are divided into the following major sections:

- An overview of the roles and functions of phlebotomists in the health care industry and the basics of anatomy and physiology with an emphasis on the circulatory system.
- Safety and infection control in the workplace and the documentation and transportation procedures needed for safe handling of biohazardous specimens.
- Equipment and procedures with the most updated questions and information about blood collection equipment.
- Special procedures and point-of-care testing, including information about pediatric phlebotomy procedures, arterial and IV collections, and special considerations for the elderly, homebound, and long-term care patients.

• Quality and legal issues, including quality management issues for blood and specimen collection services and legal issues important to phlebotomy practice.

Each chapter includes chapter objectives as a guide and an added feature of *knowledge levels* for each question. After the reader learns the essential topics in the ***Phlebotomy Handbook: Blood Collection Essentials, Fifth Edition,*** he or she can review them through the questions and answers presented in this book. Alternatively, this book may stand alone as a review book because it contains explanatory answers and the added feature of explanations for incorrect answers. These answers are all referenced to pages in the ***Phlebotomy Handbook: Blood Collection Essentials, Fifth Edition,*** so that the reader can obtain additional information on the question topic. This review book incorporates updated illustrations of blood collection equipment and techniques as bases for questions to help sharpen the phlebotomy skills. Also, a CD is included with the review book, containing color figures related to the questions and answers.

Using the book will assist the reader in identifying areas of relative strength and weakness in the command of phlebotomy skills and responsibilities. After reviewing the multiple-choice questions and answers, the reader can practice taking a simulated examination provided on the accompanying CD. A diagnostic report identifies those topics that need further review and study.

Prentice Hall Health Q&A Review for Phlebotomy, Fifth Edition, Phlebotomy Handbook: Blood Collection Essentials, Fifth Edition, and the ***Instructor's Guide*** are major *national* and *international* references for health care providers' educational programs, hospitals, physicians' offices, clinics, national examination boards, and legal issues in blood collection.

We would like to thank Susan K. Ricketts, M.Ed., CLPlb(NCA), for her thorough review of this book.

References

Garza, D. & Becan-McBride, K. (1999). *Phlebotomy Handbook: Blood Collection Essentials, Fifth Edition.* Upper Saddle River, NJ: Appleton & Lange

Kathleen Becan-McBride
Diana Garza

Introduction

 ## SUCCESS ACROSS THE BOARDS: THE PRENTICE HALL HEALTH REVIEW SERIES

Prentice Hall Health is pleased to present *Success Across the Boards,* our new review series. These authoritative texts give you expert help in preparing for certifying examinations. Each title in the series comes with its own technology package, including a CD-ROM and a Companion Website. You will find that this powerful combination of text and media provides you with expert help and guidance for achieving success across the boards.

COMPONENTS OF THE SERIES:

The series is made up of a book and CD combinations as well as a companion website that supports the book.

Q&A Review for Phlebotomy, by Kathleen Becan-McBride and Diana Garza

- *About the Book:*

- *Q&A Review for Phlebotomy, Fifth Edition:* This book has been designed to help the student prepare for the various phlebotomy certification exams. Over 650 multiple-choice questions are organized by topic areas covered on the exam and follow the exam format. For ease of reviewing the content areas, most of the quetions and answers are referenced to *Phlebotomy Handbook: Blood Collection Essentials, Fifth Edition,* by Diana Garza and Kathleen Becan-McBride. Working through these questions will help you to assess your strengths and weaknesses in each topic of study. Each question is assigned a Knowledge Level. These levels describe the cognitive skills needed to answer the questions. Knowledge Level 1 refers to *recall:* the ability to recall previously memorized knowledge skills and facts. Knowledge Level 2 refers to *applications:* the ability to apply recalled knowledge in verbal and written skills. Knowledge Level 3 refers to *problem solving:* the ability to apply recalled knowledge in solving a problem or case situation.

- *Chapter Objectives:* Each chapter includes objectives, which allow you to preview the topics covered and identify the information and skills you are responsible for knowing. These are also referenced in *Phlebotomy Handbook: Blood Collection Essentials, Fifth Edition,* by Diana Garza and Kathleen Becan-McBride, for cross-referencing and organizing studying time.
- *Answers and Rationales:* The correct answer and a rationale for it are given for every question. Rationales for each incorrect answer are provided as well so that you may learn why an answer is incorrect. Answers are referenced to the appropriate page numbers in *Phlebotomy Handbook: Blood Collection Essentials, Fifth Edition,* by Diana Garza and Kathleen Becan-McBride, for quick follow-up and additional information.
- *References:* Answers to all questions are referenced to pages in *Phlebotomy Handbook: Blood Collection Essentials, Fifth Edition,* by Diana Garza and Kathleen Becan-McBride. These references will allow you to easily find the information you need for more in-depth explanations or study on a specific topic.

- About the CD-ROM:

A CD-ROM is included in the back of this book. It includes all questions presented in the book PLUS art and illustrations. The software was designed so that you can practice by topic or through simulated exams. Correct answers and comprehensive rationales and references follow all questions. You will receive immediate feedback to identify your strengths and weaknesses in each topic covered.

- *Practice Exam:* An exam-like practice test with 100 questions is included on the CD-ROM. This test will give you a chance to experience the exam before you actually have to take it. These questions also include correct answers, rationales for correct *and* incorrect answers, and references to assist you in determining your strengths, weaknesses, and needs for further study.

Companion Website for Phlebotomy Review

Visit the companion website at *www.prenhall. com/review* for additional practice, information about the exam, and links to related resources. This site was designed as a supplement to this book in the series. You will want to bookmark it and return frequently for the most current information on your path to success.

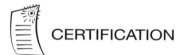

CERTIFICATION

Each of at least five organizations currently has certification tests in phlebotomy. If you intend to apply for one or more of the certification examinations, determine which particular phlebotomy certification examinations are better known and/or accepted in your local community and state.

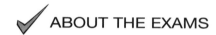

ABOUT THE EXAMS

Each organization has specific requirements for certification testing eligibility and/or continuing education requirements to maintain the certification once the examination has been passed. Requirements are subject to change or revisions periodically, so you need to contact the associations directly to inquire about your specific qualifications and experience. Plan ahead of time to find out about the testing requirements and the testing location, date, and time that most suits you.

American Society of Clinical Pathologists (ASCP)
2100 W. Harrison St.
Chicago, IL 60612
(312) 738-1336 or (800) 621-4142
E-mail: info@ascp.org
Website: www.ascp.org

American Medical Technologists (AMT)
710 Higgins Rd., Park Ridge, IL 60068
(847) 823-5169 or (800) 275-1268
E-mail: AMTMAIL@aol.com
Website: www.AMT1.com

American Society of Phlebotomy Technicians (ASPT)
1109 2nd Ave. S.W., P.O. Box 1831
Hickory, NC 28603
(828) 322-1334
E-mail: aspt@abts.net
Website: www.aspt.org

National Phlebotomy Association (NPA)
1901 Brightseat Road
Landover, MD 20785
(301) 386-4200
E-mail: npa78@aol.com

National Credentialing Agency (NCA)
P.O. Box 15945-289, Lenexa, KS 66285
(913) 438-5110, ext. 487
E-mail: NCA-INFO@applmeapro.com
Website: www.applmeapro.com/nca/

Information about examinations may change, so be sure to obtain current information by contacting the examination boards.

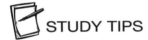 STUDY TIPS

Review Materials

Choose review materials that contain the information you need to study. Save time by making sure that you are not studying anything you do not need to. The best preparation before the exam is to work through the questions in this review book to determine your strengths and weaknesses. The page references at the end of each answer will direct you to sections in *Phlebotomy Handbook: Blood Collection Essentials, Fifth Edition,* so that you can obtain additional information on the question topic.

Set a Study Schedule

Use your time management skills to set a schedule that will help you feel as prepared as you can be. Consider all the relevant factors: the materials you need to study; how many months, weeks, or days until the test date; and how much time you can study each day. If you establish your schedule ahead of time and write it in your date book, you will be much more likely to follow it.

Take Practice Tests

Practice as much as possible, using the questions in this book, on the accompanying CD-ROM, and on the companion website. These questions were designed to follow the format of questions that appear on the exam you will take, so the more you practice with these questions, the better prepared you will be on test day.

The printed practice tests in the book and on the CD-ROM will give you a chance to experience the exam before you actually have to take it and will also let you know how you're doing and where you need to do better. For best results, we recommend that you take a practice test 2 to 3 weeks before you are scheduled to take the actual exam. Spend the next weeks targeting the areas in which you performed poorly and practice additional questions in those areas.

Practice under testlike conditions: in a quiet room, with no books or notes to help you, and with a clock telling you when to quit. Try to come as close as you can to duplicating the actual test situation.

TAKING THE EXAMINATION

Prepare Physically

When taking the exam, you need to work efficiently under time pressure. If your body is tired or under stress, you might not think as clearly or perform as well as you usually do. If you can, avoid staying up all night. Get some sleep so that you can wake up rested and alert.

Eating right is also important. The best advice is to eat a light, well-balanced meal before a test. When time is short, grab a quick-energy snack such as a banana, orange juice, or a granola bar.

The Examination Site

The examination site must be located before the required examination time. One suggestion is to find the site and parking facilities the day before the test. Parking fee information should be obtained ahead of time so that sufficient money can be taken along on the examination day.

Allow plenty of time for travel to the site in case of unexpected mishaps such as traffic snarls. During travel, think positive thoughts (e.g., "My preparation for the exam was thorough, so I'll be able to answer the questions easily"). Maintain a confident attitude to prevent unnecessary stress.

Materials

Be sure to take all required identification materials, registration forms, and any other items required by the testing organization or center. Thoroughly read information and instructions supplied by the testing organizations to be sure you have all necessary materials before the day of the exam.

Read Test Directions

Read the examination directions thoroughly! Because some board examinations have different test sections with different question formats, it is important to be aware of changes in directions. Read each set of directions completely before starting a new section of questions.

Machine-scored tests require that you use a special pencil to fill in a small box on a computerized answer sheet. Use the right pencil (usually a number 2), and mark your answers in the correct space. Neatness counts on these tests because the computer can misread stray pencil marks or partially erased answers. Periodically, check the answer number against the question number to make sure they match. One question skipped can cause every answer following it to be marked incorrectly.

Selecting the Right Answer

Keep in mind that only one answer is correct. First read the stem of the question with *each* possible choice provided, and eliminate choices that are obviously incorrect. Be cautious about choosing the first answer that *might* be correct; all possibilities should be considered before the final choice is made; the best answer should be selected.

If a question is complicated, try to break it down into small sections that are easy to understand. Pay special attention to qualifiers such as *only, except,* and the like. For example, negative words in a question can confuse your understanding of what the question asks ("Which of the following is *not . . .* ").

Intelligent Guessing

If you don't know the answer, eliminate those answers that you know or suspect are wrong. Your goal is to narrow down your choices. Here are some questions to ask yourself:

- Is the choice accurate in its own terms? If there is an error in the choice—for example, a term that is incorrectly defined—the answer is wrong.
- Is the choice relevant? An answer may be accurate, but it might not relate to the essence of the question.
- Are there any qualifiers, such as *always, never, all, none,* or *every?* Qualifiers make it easy to find an exception that makes a choice incorrect.

Mark answers you aren't sure of, and go back to them at the end of the test.

Ask yourself whether you would make the same guesses again. Chances are that you will leave your answers alone, but you may notice something that will make you change your mind—a qualifier that affects meaning or a remembered fact that will enable you to answer the question without guessing.

Watch the Clock

Keep track of how much time is left and how you are progressing. Wear a watch or bring a small clock with you to the test room. A wall clock may be broken, or there may be no clock at all.

Some students are so concerned about time that they rush through the exam and have time left over. In such situations, it's easy to leave early. The best approach, however, is to take your time. Stay until the end so that you can check your answers.

Computerized Exams

To ensure that you are comfortable with the computer test format, be sure to practice on the computer, using the CD-ROM that is included in the back of this book.

Since certification exam requirements vary, it is important to determine before taking a computerized exam whether you can change your answer after you strike a key for a particular answer. Checking your answers is a very important part of taking a major certification exam. Thus do not enter an answer on a computerized exam unless you (1) have the option to change it as you are checking your answers or (2) are absolutely certain that your answer is correct when you first enter it.

During the exam, check the computer screen after an answer is entered to verify that the answer appears as it was entered. If you feel fatigued, close your eyes, take a few deep breaths, and stretch your arms and shoulders; then resume the examination.

KEYS TO SUCCESS ACROSS THE BOARD

- Study, review, and practice
- Keep a positive, confident attitude
- Follow all directions on the examination
- Do your best

Good luck!

You are encouraged to visit http://www.prenhall. com/success *for additional tips on studying, test taking, and other keys to success. At this stage of your education and career, you will find these tips helpful.*

Some of the study and test-taking tips were adapted from Keys to Effective Learning, Second Edition, *by Carol Carter, Joyce Bishop, and Sarah Lyman Kravits.*

SECTION I

Overview

1

1 Phlebotomy Practice and Health Care Settings

chapter objectives

Upon completion of Chapter 1, the learner is responsible for the following:

➤ Define phlebotomy practice and list the essential competencies for individuals performing phlebotomy/blood collection procedures.

➤ Identify health care providers who generally perform phlebotomy procedures.

➤ Identify the importance of phlebotomy procedures to the overall care of the patient.

➤ List skills for active listening and effective verbal communication.

➤ List examples of positive and negative body language.

➤ Describe various health care settings, both inpatient and ambulatory, where phlebotomy services are routinely performed.

➤ Describe the role of the clinical laboratory in blood collection and testing services.

DIRECTIONS Each of the questions or incomplete statements below is followed by four suggested answers or completions. Select **one answer** that is best in each case.

 KNOWLEDGE LEVEL = 2

1. In the clinical chemistry area, which of the following assays is usually performed?
   A. total proteins
   B. cold agglutinins
   C. rheumatoid factor
   D. ABO grouping

 KNOWLEDGE LEVEL = 1

2. In the clinical laboratory, the abbreviation CSF is used for:
   A. clinical serum fluid
   B. cerebrospinal fluid
   C. cerebral serum fluid
   D. clinical spinal fluid

 KNOWLEDGE LEVEL = 3

3. Which of the following assays is included in the routine UA?
   A. triglycerides
   B. Coombs' test
   C. RPR
   D. urobilinogen

 KNOWLEDGE LEVEL = 2

4. The clinical laboratory department usually includes:
   A. clinical pharmacy
   B. anatomic pathology
   C. clinical encephalography
   D. diagnostic imaging

 KNOWLEDGE LEVEL = 1

5. The health care institutional department that uses radioactive isotopes or tracers in the diagnosis and treatment of patients and in the study of the disease process is the:
   A. clinical laboratory department
   B. occupational therapy department
   C. nuclear medicine department
   D. diagnostic imaging/radiology department

 KNOWLEDGE LEVEL = 1

6. Which of the following medical departments is associated with diagnostic and treatment procedures for bone and joint disorders and diseases?
   A. dermatology
   B. orthopedics
   C. ophthalmology
   D. otolaryngology

 KNOWLEDGE LEVEL = 1

7. Which of the following departments that are found in most large health care facilities deals with the general diagnosis and treatment of patients for problems of one or more internal organs?
   A. anesthesiology
   B. proctology
   C. internal medicine
   D. oncology

KNOWLEDGE LEVEL = 1

8. Which of the following clinical laboratory sections usually has drug analysis?
   A. clinical microbiology
   B. clinical chemistry
   C. clinical immunology
   D. hematology

 KNOWLEDGE LEVEL = 2

9. Which of the following analytes is a hormone?
   A. cortisol
   B. cholesterol
   C. HDL cholesterol
   D. blood urea nitrogen

 KNOWLEDGE LEVEL = 1

10. Which of the following requires a two-year certificate or associate degree in the study of laboratory testing and procedures, preparing specimens for testing and transport, and performing quality-control measures?
    A. MLT
    B. MT
    C. CLS
    D. pathologist

 KNOWLEDGE LEVEL = 1

11. Of the following personnel, which health care worker is sometimes referred to as a clinical laboratory technician?
    A. medical technologist
    B. phlebotomist
    C. clinical laboratory scientist
    D. MLT

 KNOWLEDGE LEVEL = 1

12. A primary consultant on drug therapy is found in which of the following departments?
    A. occupational therapy
    B. clinical laboratory
    C. pharmacy
    D. nutrition and dietetics

 KNOWLEDGE LEVEL = 2

13. Which of the following procedures is usually considered primary care?
    A. immunizations
    B. CAT scan
    C. ophthalmology examination
    D. open-heart surgery

 KNOWLEDGE LEVEL = 1

14. To become a medical technologist requires which of the following degrees at a minimum?
    A. associate's
    B. bachelor's
    C. master's
    D. doctorate

 KNOWLEDGE LEVEL = 1

15. A physician who usually has extensive education in the study and diagnosis of diseases through the use of laboratory test results is sometimes referred to as a:
    A. medical technologist
    B. pathologist
    C. medical laboratory technician
    D. clinical laboratory scientist

KNOWLEDGE LEVEL = 1

16. Which of the following departments deals with disorders affecting the organs and tissues that produce hormones?
    A. nephrology
    B. neurology
    C. endocrinology
    D. otolaryngology

 KNOWLEDGE LEVEL = 2

17. Employers of health care workers are legally required to provide PPE for workers, which includes:
    A. bar code labels for patients' specimens
    B. face shields
    C. BD Unopettes
    D. Velcro-type tourniquets

 KNOWLEDGE LEVEL = 1

18. Which of the following departments is involved in the diagnosis and treatment of malignant tumors?
    A. rheumatology
    B. geriatrics
    C. proctology
    D. oncology

 KNOWLEDGE LEVEL = 1

19. Medicare, which is used frequently in health care services, refers to a:
    A. joint federal and state program covering health services for the poor and other special populations
    B. federal program covering health services for the elderly
    C. federal government regulation over all clinical laboratory testing

    D. joint federal and state program to regulate all clinical laboratories for complexity of laboratory testing procedures

 KNOWLEDGE LEVEL = 1

20. The department of gastroenterology refers to:
    A. organs and tissues that produce hormones
    B. ears, nose, and throat
    C. esophagus, stomach, and intestines
    D. nervous system

 KNOWLEDGE LEVEL = 2

21. Mrs. J. Hamm, a patient who had blood tests requested from the nephrology department, probably has a disorder related to the:
    A. nervous system
    B. lungs
    C. immune system
    D. kidneys

 KNOWLEDGE LEVEL = 2

22. The AHA Patient's Bill of Rights has key elements including:
    A. Medicaid eligibility
    B. Medicare eligibility
    C. informed consent
    D. personal protective equipment

 KNOWLEDGE LEVEL = 1

23. From the following, who is considered a health care specialist?
    A. physician assistant
    B. nurse practitioner
    C. nurse midwife
    D. ophthalmologist

KNOWLEDGE LEVEL = 1

24. Ambulatory care refers to health care services provided to:
    A. outpatients
    B. inpatients
    C. patients in acute care hospitals
    D. patients in long-term care hospitals

 KNOWLEDGE LEVEL = 3

25. Which of the following is *not* an important purpose of laboratory analyses to the entire health assessment on a patient?
    A. monitoring of the patient's health status
    B. therapeutic assessment to develop the appropriate treatment
    C. monitoring of the patient's health status to develop a community needs assessment
    D. diagnostic testing on the patient

 KNOWLEDGE LEVEL = 2

26. On the basis of recommended professional competencies for a board-certified phlebotomist, which of the following is a phlebotomist's professional competency?
    A. selects appropriate quality control procedures
    B. performs microscopic analysis of blood smears
    C. participates in the development of new laboratory testing instrumentation
    D. performs tests and records immunologic laboratory procedural results.

 KNOWLEDGE LEVEL = 3

27. The federal government regulates *all* clinical laboratories through:
    A. Medicare
    B. Medicaid

C. CLIA 1988
D. American Association of Blood Banks

 KNOWLEDGE LEVEL = 2

28. In which of the following departments is it extremely important for the phlebotomist to be knowledgeable of special safety requirements for entering this area?
    A. electrocardiography department
    B. nuclear medicine department
    C. occupational therapy department
    D. nutrition and dietetics department

 KNOWLEDGE LEVEL = 1

29. The laboratory test referred to as BUN is an abbreviation for:
    A. blood uric nitrogen
    B. blood urea nitrogen
    C. bilirubin urea nitrogen
    D. bilirubin uric nitrogen

 KNOWLEDGE LEVEL = 2

30. The terms pH, PCO_2, and PO_2 are used in the testing of:
    A. blood urea nitrogen
    B. electrolytes
    C. blood gases
    D. enzymes

 KNOWLEDGE LEVEL = 1

31. Rh phenotyping and genotyping occur in:
    A. clinical immunology
    B. immunohematology
    C. clinical microscopy
    D. hematology

KNOWLEDGE LEVEL = 2

32. The clinical laboratory supervisor requested that Ms. Douglas, a phlebotomist, go quickly to the otolaryngology department to pick up a laboratory specimen on Ms. Gonzales. The phlebotomist had to go to the department that provides treatment of the:
    A. skin
    B. eyes
    C. bones and joints
    D. ears, nose, and throat

 KNOWLEDGE LEVEL = 1

33. When there is a referral to specialized care involving a physician who is an expert on a particular group of diseases, a group of organ systems, or an organ, this type of care is:
    A. primary care
    B. secondary care
    C. tertiary care
    D. quaternary care

 KNOWLEDGE LEVEL = 2

34. Which of the following is appropriate protocol for health care workers who are involved in specimen collection?
    A. Once the laboratory tests have been performed on a patient, the blood collector can discuss these with the patient and family.
    B. If the family asked for information on their child's laboratory results, the blood collector should seek those results out to help the family.
    C. The blood collector should state that the patient's physician ordered blood to be collected for testing and that it would be best to discuss the laboratory tests with the physician.

    D. If the blood collector is a phlebotomy student, it is best not to inform the patient that he or she is a student, since it may make the patient nervous.

 KNOWLEDGE LEVEL = 1

35. If the phlebotomist collects blood in the neonatology department, he or she is performing blood collection on patients who are:
    A. zero to a few days old
    B. one to three years old
    C. ready to have a baby
    D. three to five years old

 KNOWLEDGE LEVEL = 2

36. Which of the following is a term used for a health care worker who has patient care duties along with specimen collection duties?
    A. occupational therapist
    B. physical therapist
    C. clinical laboratory scientist
    D. patient care technician

 KNOWLEDGE LEVEL = 3

37. For CLIA 88 regulatory categories, which of the following are designated in the waivered tests category?
    A. urine cultures
    B. urinalysis
    C. bone marrow evaluation
    D. cytogenetics

KNOWLEDGE LEVEL = 1

38. CBC is an abbreviation for:
    A. complete blood cells
    B. complete blood count
    C. cerebrospinal blood count
    D. cerebrospinal blood cells

KNOWLEDGE LEVEL = 2

39. Blood that is collected for the salicylates level is usually taken to what clinical laboratory section for testing?
    A. hematology
    B. clinical immunology
    C. immunohematology
    D. clinical chemistry

KNOWLEDGE LEVEL = 2

40. Blood for the LE cell preparation is usually taken to what clinical laboratory section for testing?
    A. hematology
    B. clinical immunology
    C. immunohematology
    D. clinical chemistry

KNOWLEDGE LEVEL = 2

41. Blood for which of the following procedures should be taken to the clinical chemistry section of the clinical laboratory?
    A. hemoglobin
    B. CBC
    C. glycated hemoglobin
    D. hematocrit

KNOWLEDGE LEVEL = 1

42. Which of the following should the phlebotomist avoid in his or her patient care and blood collection activities?
    A. making eye contact with the patient
    B. making a deep sigh when collecting the blood
    C. smiling when he or she is around the patient
    D. maintaining relaxed hands, arms, and shoulders

KNOWLEDGE LEVEL = 1

43. Which of the following is *not* considered to be an ambulatory care setting?
    A. community health center
    B. veteran's hospital
    C. physician group practice
    D. hospital-based clinic

KNOWLEDGE LEVEL = 1

44. Which of the following departments in health care facilities has the specific responsibilities with diagnosis and treatment of the elderly population?
    A. psychiatry/neurology
    B. geriatrics
    C. internal medicine
    D. proctology

KNOWLEDGE LEVEL = 1

45. Which of the following departments in health care facilities has the specific responsibility of correcting the deformity of tissues, including skin?
    A. proctology
    B. physical medicine
    C. plastic surgery
    D. psychiatry/neurology

KNOWLEDGE LEVEL = 2

46. Which of the following patients' specimens would most likely be taken to anatomic pathology?
    A. cerebrospinal fluid
    B. sputum
    C. synovial fluid
    D. biopsy tissue

KNOWLEDGE LEVEL = 2

47. Ms. Pickins, a 24-year-old phlebotomist at High Island Hospital, is in her third month of pregnancy. Which of the following sections or departments of the hospital should she avoid for any blood collections or pick-ups for transportation to the laboratory?
    A. encephalography section
    B. radiotherapy section
    C. physical therapy department
    D. pharmacy department

 KNOWLEDGE LEVEL = 3

48. According to the Clinical Laboratory Improvement Amendments of 1988 (CLIA 88), the electrophoresis test is considered to be a:
    A. waivered test
    B. moderate-complexity test
    C. high-complexity test
    D. extremely high-complexity test

 KNOWLEDGE LEVEL = 3

49. Follow-up treatment of chronic illnesses and diseases such as diabetes mellitus is frequently provided through:
    A. primary health care services
    B. secondary health care services
    C. tertiary health care services
    D. quaternary health care services

 KNOWLEDGE LEVEL = 2

50. As a phlebotomist, you have a STAT blood specimen to be collected on Mr. Tsu for the Legionnaires' disease antibody. Which section of the clinical laboratory will perform the test on this blood specimen?
    A. clinical microscopy
    B. clinical immunology/serology
    C. hematology and coagulation
    D. immunohematology

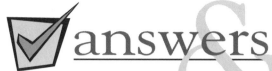

answers & rationales

1.

A. The total proteins assay is generally performed in the clinical chemistry area of the laboratory. (p. 34)

B. The cold agglutinins assay is usually performed in the clinical immunology area of the laboratory.

C. The rheumatoid factor assay is usually performed in the clinical immunology area of the laboratory.

D. ABO grouping is performed in the immunohematology (blood bank or transfusion medicine) area of the clinical laboratory.

2.

A. CSF is the abbreviation used for cerebrospinal fluid, not clinical serum fluid.

B. CSF is the abbreviation used for cerebrospinal fluid. (p. 35)

C. CSF is the abbreviation used for cerebrospinal fluid, not cerebral serum fluid.

D. CSF is the abbreviation used for cerebrospinal fluid, not clinical spinal fluid.

3.

A. The triglycerides assay is usually performed in the chemistry area.

B. The Coombs' test is performed in the immunohematology (blood bank or transfusion medicine) area.

C. The RPR test is usually performed in the clinical immunology area.

D. The urobilinogen assay is included in the routine urinalysis (UA). (p. 35)

4.

A. The clinical pharmacy department dispenses medications ordered by physicians. It is not part of the clinical laboratory department.

B. Anatomic pathology and clinical pathology are the two major components of the typical hospital-based clinical laboratory. (p. 30)

C. Clinical encephalography uses the electroencephalogram (EEG) to record brain wave patterns. It is not part of the clinical laboratory.

D. Diagnostic imaging uses ionizing radiation for treating diseases. It is not part of the clinical laboratory.

5.

A. The clinical laboratory department uses instrumentation to analyze blood, body fluids and tissues for pathological conditions.

B. The occupational therapy department assists the patient in becoming functionally independent within the limitations of the patient's disability or condition.

C. The nuclear medicine department uses radioactive isotopes or tracers in the diagnosis and treatment of patients and in the study of the disease process. (p. 31)

D. The diagnostic imaging/radiology department uses ionizing radiation for treating disease, fluoroscopic and radiographic x-ray instrumentation and imaging for diagnosis and treating disease.

6.

A. Dermatology is the department that has medical treatments for skin disorders.

B. The orthopedics department performs diagnostic and treatment procedures for bone and joint disorders and diseases. (p. 30)

C. Ophthalmology is the department that has medical diagnosis and treatment for eye disorders.

D. Otolaryngology is the department that has medical diagnosis and treatment for ear, nose, and throat disorders.

7.

A. Ophthalmology is the department that has medical diagnosis and treatment for eye disorders.

B. Otolaryngology is the department that has medical diagnosis and treatment for ear, nose, and throat disorders.

C. Internal medicine is the department involved in the general diagnosis and treatment of patients for problems of one or more internal organs. (p. 29)

D. Oncology is the department involved in the diagnosis and treatment of malignant tumors.

8.

A. The clinical microbiology department performs analyses to detect microorganisms that are infecting the patient and include such tests as occult blood, blood cultures, and strep screening.

B. Clinical chemistry is the section that performs analyses on drugs such as gentamicin, tobramycin, digoxin, salicylates, blood alcohol, and barbiturates. (p. 34)

C. The clinical immunology section performs analyses to detect antibodies and antigens that appear in the bloodstream of a patient infected with certain microorganisms.

D. The hematology section performs analyses on blood to detect abnormal types and numbers of blood cells.

9.

A. Cortisol is a hormone secreted from the adrenal gland, and its blood level is analyzed in the clinical chemistry section. (p. 34)

B. Cholesterol is not a hormone, but rather a lipid (fat) that is measured in the blood.

C. HDL cholesterol is not a hormone, but rather a type of lipid (fat) that has been determined to be "good" for a person. Its blood level is usually measured in the clinical chemistry section.

D. Blood urea nitrogen (BUN) is not a hormone but rather a blood waste product from the breakdown of proteins in the body.

10.

A. The medical laboratory technician (MLT) requires a two-year certificate or associate degree in the study of laboratory testing and procedures, preparing specimens for testing and transport, and performing quality-control measures. (p. 32)

B. The medical technologist (MT) or clinical laboratory scientist (CLS) is an individual who has a bachelor's degree in a biological science, including at least one year in the study of clinical laboratory sciences.

C. The medical technologist (MT) or clinical laboratory scientist (CLS) is an individual who has a bachelor's degree in a biological science, including at least one year in the study of clinical laboratory sciences.

D. The pathologist is a physician who has extensive training in the study and diagnosis of disease through the use of laboratory test results.

11.

A. The medical technologist (MT) or clinical laboratory scientist (CLS) requires a baccalaureate degree in biological sciences with at least one year devoted to the study of clinical laboratory sciences.

B. The phlebotomist is also referred to as the blood collector and performs blood collection and transports specimens to the laboratory testing area.

C. The medical technologist (MT) or clinical laboratory scientist (CLS) requires a baccalaureate degree in biological sciences with at least one year devoted to the study of clinical laboratory sciences.

D. The clinical laboratory technician (CLT) or medical laboratory technician (MLT) requires a two-year certificate or associate degree in the study of laboratory testing, procedures, and quality-control measures. (p. 32)

12.

A. The occupational therapy department assists the patient in becoming functionally independent within the limitations of the patient's disability or condition.

B. The clinical laboratory department uses sophisticated instrumentation to analyze blood, body fluids, and tissues for pathological conditions.

C. The pharmacy department dispenses medications ordered by the physician and collaborates with the health care team on drug therapies. (p. 31)

D. The nutrition and dietetics department performs nutritional assessments, patient education and designs special diets for patients who have eating-related disorders.

13.

A. Primary care is given to maintain and monitor normal health and to prevent diseases by means of immunizations and laboratory screening tests. (p. 27)

B. The computer axial tomography (CAT) scan is a very sophisticated instrument that is used to make complex diagnoses in tertiary care.

C. The ophthalmology exam is given to diagnose and treat eye disorders and is considered specialized secondary health care.

D. Open-heart surgery is a very complex type of tertiary care.

14.

A. To become a medical laboratory technician (MLT) requires an associate degree in clinical laboratory testing and procedures. However, a MT requires a bachelor's degree.

B. To become a medical technologist requires a bachelor's degree in biological sciences with at least one year of study in clinical laboratory sciences. (p. 31)

C. To become a medical technologist requires a bachelor's degree in biological sciences with at least one year of study in clinical laboratory sciences.

D. To become a medical technologist requires a bachelor's degree in biological sciences with at least one year of study in clinical laboratory sciences.

15.

A. A medical technologist (MT) has a bachelor's degree in a biological science with at least one year of study in a clinical laboratory science program.

B. A pathologist is a physician who has extensive training in pathology, which is the study and diagnosis of diseases through the use of laboratory test results. (p. 30)

C. A medical laboratory technician (MLT) has an associate's degree in the study of clinical laboratory testing and procedures.

D. A clinical laboratory scientist (CLS) is a medical technologist who has a bachelor's degree in a biological science with at least one year of study in a clinical laboratory science program.

16.

A. The nephrology department deals with renal (kidney) system disorders.

B. The neurology department deals with nervous system disorders.

C. The endocrinology department deals with disorders affecting organs and tissues that produce hormones. (p. 30)

D. The otolaryngology department deals with disorders of the ear, nose, and throat.

17.

A. PPE is personal protective equipment, and bar code labels for patients' specimens do not fit the definition.

B. Employers of health care workers are legally required to provide personal protective equipment (PPE) such as face shields and gowns. (p. 25)

C. BD Unopettes (BD VACUTAINER Systems, Franklin Lakes, NJ) are used for microcollection of blood. They are *not* personal protective equipment (PPE).

D. Velcro-type tourniquets are used to place around a patient's arm for venipuncture. They are *not* personal protective equipment (PPE) for the health care worker.

18.

A. Rheumatology is the department involved in the diagnosis and treatment of joint and tissue diseases, including arthritis.

B. Geriatrics is the department involved in the diagnosis and treatment of the elderly population.

C. Proctology is the department involved in the diagnosis and treatment of diseases of the anus and rectum.

D. Oncology is the department involved in the diagnosis and treatment of malignant (life-threatening) tumors. (p. 29)

19.

A. Medicaid, not Medicare, is a joint federal and state program covering health services for the poor and other special populations.

B. Medicare is a federal program covering health services for the elderly. (p. 28)

C. The federal government has a regulatory program over all clinical laboratory testing referred to as CLIA, not Medicare.

D. Medicare is a federal program covering health services for the elderly.

20.

A. The department of endocrinology deals with disorders and diseases of the organs and tissues that produce hormones.

B. The department of otolaryngology deals with disorders and diseases of the ears, nose, and throat.

C. The department of gastroenterology deals with diseases and disorders related to the esophagus, stomach, and intestines. (p. 30)

D. The neurology department deals with disorders and diseases of the nervous system.

21.

A. The department of neurology deals with disorders and diseases of the nervous system.

B. The pulmonary division deals with disorders and diseases of the lungs.

C. Immunology is the department that deals with disorders and diseases of the immune system.

D. The nephrology department deals with disorders and diseases of the kidneys. (p. 30)

22.

A. Medicaid eligibility is a federal and state program for health services for the poor and is not part of the AHA Patient's Bill of Rights.

B. Medicare eligibility is a federal program for health services for the elderly and is not part of the AHA Patient's Bill of Rights.

C. The AHA Patient's Bill of Rights has several key elements including informed consent. (p. 25)

D. Personal protective equipment (PPE) is required for health care workers by their employers under federal regulations and not under the AHA Patient's Bill of Rights.

23.

A. A physician assistant is considered a primary health care worker.

B. A nurse practitioner is considered a primary health care worker.

C. A nurse midwife is considered a primary health care worker.

D. The ophthalmologist is a physician who provides specialized health care for the eyes. (pp. 27, 30)

24.

A. Ambulatory care refers to personal health care provided to an individual who is not bedridden and therefore is an outpatient. (p. 28)

B. Ambulatory care refers to personal health care provided to an individual who is not bedridden.

C. Ambulatory care refers to personal health care provided to an individual who is not bedridden.

D. Ambulatory care refers to personal health care provided to an individual who is not bedridden.

25.

A. Monitoring of the patient's health status through laboratory analysis is used to make sure the therapy of treatment is working to alleviate the medical condition.

B. Therapeutic assessment through laboratory analysis is used to develop the appropriate therapy of treatment of the medical condition for the patient.

C. Monitoring of the patient's health status to develop a community needs assessment can be very helpful to the overall community but sometimes does not fit the immediate monitoring needs for the entire health assessment through laboratory analysis on a particular patient. (p. 7)

D. Clinical laboratory technicians and clinical laboratory scientists perform tests and record immunologic laboratory procedures.

26.

A. The phlebotomist is constantly involved in selecting the appropriate quality control procedures such as monitoring the expiration dates on blood collection vacuum tubes. (p. 9)

B. Clinical laboratory scientists perform the microscopic analysis of blood smears whereas the phlebotomist collects the blood smears for the microscopic analysis.

C. Clinical laboratory scientists participate in the development of new laboratory testing instrumentation.

D. Clinical laboratory technicians and clinical laboratory scientists perform tests and record immunologic laboratory procedures.

27.

A. Medicare, a federal program covering health services for the elderly has oversight only of clinical laboratories that participate in Medicare reimbursement.

B. Medicaid, a federal and state program covering health services for the poor and other special populations, has oversight only of clinical laboratories that participate in Medicaid reimbursement.

C. The federal government regulates all clinical laboratories through the Clinical Laboratory Improvement Amendments of 1988 (CLIA 1988). (p. 33)

D. The American Association of Blood Banks (AABB) has oversight only of clinical laboratories that have blood banking (transfusion medicine testing).

28.

A. The nuclear medicine department uses radioactive isotopes or tracers in the diagnosis and treatment of patients and the radioisotopes may interfere with laboratory testing.

B. The nuclear medicine department uses radioactive isotopes or tracers in the diagnosis and treatment of patients, and the radioisotopes may interfere with laboratory testing. (p. 31)

C. The nuclear medicine department uses radioactive isotopes or tracers in the diagnosis and treatment of patients and the radioisotopes may interfere with laboratory testing.

D. The nuclear medicine department uses radioactive isotopes or tracers in the diagnosis and treatment of patients and the radioisotopes may interfere with laboratory testing.

29.

A. The laboratory test referred to as BUN is an abbreviation for blood urea nitrogen.

B. The laboratory test referred to as BUN is an abbreviation for blood urea nitrogen. (p. 34)

C. The laboratory test referred to as BUN is an abbreviation for blood urea nitrogen.

D. The laboratory test referred to as BUN is an abbreviation for blood urea nitrogen.

30.

A. Blood urea nitrogen is not the testing of pH, pCO_2, and pO_2, but rather urea nitrogen in the blood.

B. Electrolytes measure sodium, potassium, chloride, and bicarbonate in the blood.

C. Blood gases (pH, partial pressure of carbon dioxide [pCO_2], and partial pressure of oxygen [pO_2]) are measured on arterial or capillary blood. (p. 34)

D. Enzymes measure lactate dehydrogenase, creatine phosphokinase, alanine aminotransferase, and others, but pH, pCO_2, and pO_2 are not enzymes.

31.

A. Rh phenotyping and genotyping occur in the immunohematology section of the clinical laboratory.

B. Rh phenotyping and genotyping occur in the immunohematology section of the clinical laboratory. (p. 35)

C. Rh phenotyping and genotyping occur in the immunohematology section of the clinical laboratory.

D. Rh phenotyping and genotyping occur in the immunohematology section of the clinical laboratory.

32.

A. Skin diseases and disorders are treated in the dermatology department.

B. Eye diseases and disorders are treated in the ophthalmology department.

C. Bone and joint diseases and disorders are treated in the orthopedics department.

D. The otolaryngology department is involved in the diagnosis and treatment of disorders and diseases related to the ears, nose, and throat. (p. 30)

33.

A. Primary care involves treatment of minor injuries and diagnosis and treatment of colds or sore throats.

B. Secondary care involves specialized care from a physician who is an expert on a particular group of diseases, a group of organ systems, or an organ. (p. 27)

C. Tertiary care is highly specialized and oriented toward unusual and complex diagnoses and therapies.

D. There is no such term as quarternary care.

34.

A. The blood collector should state that the patient's physician ordered blood to be collected for testing and that it would be best to discuss the laboratory test with the physician.

B. The blood collector should state that the patient's physician ordered blood to be collected for testing and that it would be best to discuss the laboratory test with the physician.

C. The blood collector should state that the patient's physician ordered blood to be collected for testing and that it would be best to discuss the laboratory test with the physician. (p. 26)

D. The blood collector should state that the patient's physician ordered blood to be collected for testing and that it would be best to discuss the laboratory test with the physician.

35.

A. The neonatology department treats and supports the needs of newborn and prematurely born babies. (p. 29)

B. The neonatology department treats and supports the needs of newborn and prematurely born babies.

C. The neonatology department treats and supports the needs of newborn and prematurely born babies.

D. The neonatology department treats and supports the needs of newborn and prematurely born babies.

36.

A. Occupational therapists work in rehabilitation centers or hospitals to improve the functional abilities of patients. They do not have specimen collection duties.

B. Physical therapists assist patients in restoring physical abilities that have been impaired by illness or injury. However, they do not have specimen collection duties.

C. Clinical laboratory scientists perform laboratory tests and operate sophisticated instruments for testing patients' specimens. They are not involved in patient care duties but may occasionally collect blood specimens.

D. The patient care technician or clinical assistant is a recently added job title that integrates specimen collection duties with patient care duties. (p. 27)

37.

A. Urine cultures are categorized as a moderate-complexity test owing to the risk to the patient if results are inaccurate.

B. Waivered tests are those tests that are easiest to perform and least risky to patients. They include urinalysis. (p. 33)

C. A bone marrow evaluation is a high-complexity test because it can lead to a reasonable risk of harm to the patient if results are inaccurate.

D. Cytogenetics is the category of high-complexity testing because it can lead to a reasonable risk of harm to the patient if results are inaccurate.

38. (B)

A. CBC is an abbreviation for "complete blood count."

B. CBC is an abbreviation for "complete blood count." (p. 35)

C. CBC is an abbreviation for "complete blood count"

D. CBC is an abbreviation for "complete blood count."

39.

A. Drug analysis, including salicylates level, are usually tested in the clinical chemistry section of the clinical laboratory.

B. Drug analysis, including salicylates level, are usually tested in the clinical chemistry section of the clinical laboratory.

C. Drug analysis, including salicylates level, are usually tested in the clinical chemistry section of the clinical laboratory.

D. Drug analysis, including salicylates level, are usually tested in the clinical chemistry section of the clinical laboratory. (p. 34)

40.

A. The LE (lupus erythematosus) cell preparation is usually tested in the hematology section of the clinical laboratory. (p. 34)

B. The LE (lupus erythematosus) cell preparation is usually tested in the hematology section of the clinical laboratory.

C. The LE (lupus erythematosus) cell preparation is usually tested in the hematology section of the clinical laboratory.

D. The LE (lupus erythematosus) cell preparation is usually tested in the hematology section of the clinical laboratory.

41.

A. Blood for the hemoglobin procedure should be transported to the hematology section.

B. Blood for the CBC should be taken to the hematology section.

C. Blood for the glycated hemoglobin procedure should be taken to the clinical chemistry section. (p. 34)

D. Blood for the hematocrit test should be taken to the hematology section.

42.

A. Making eye contact with the patient should *not* be avoided. It conveys a sense of trust

B. The phlebotomist should avoid making deep sighs around patients, since this can convey a feeling of being bored. (p. 23)

C. A smile should not be avoided, since it makes the patient feel important.

D. Maintaining relaxed hands, arms, and shoulders during blood collection shows that the phlebotomist has confidence and reassurance in his or her responsibilities.

43.

A. The community health center is an ambulatory care setting, since health care is provided to individuals who are not bedridden.

B. Ambulatory care is personal health care that is provided to an individual who is not bedridden, whereas a veteran's hospital has many bedridden patients. (p. 28)

C. A physician group practice is an ambulatory care setting, since health care is provided to individuals who are not bedridden.

D. A hospital-based clinic is an ambulatory care setting, since health care is provided to individuals who are not bedridden.

44.

A. Psychiatry/neurology is the department that is involved in the diagnosis and treatment for people of all ages with mental, emotional, and nervous system problems.

B. Geriatrics is the department that is specifically responsible for the diagnosis and treatment of the elderly population. (p. 29)

C. Internal medicine is a health care facility department that is involved in the general diagnosis and treatment of patients for problems of one or more internal organs.

D. Proctology is the department in the health care facility that is involved in the diagnosis and treatment of diseases of the anus and rectum.

45.

A. Proctology is the department in health care facilities that is involved in the diagnosis and treatment of diseases of the anus and rectum.

B. The department of physical medicine takes care of the diagnosis and treatment of disorders and disabilities of the neuromuscular system.

C. Plastic surgery is the department in health care facilities that oversees the correction of the deformity of tissues including skin. (p. 29)

D. The department of psychiatry/neurology handles the diagnosis and treatment of people with mental, emotional, and nervous system problems.

46.

A. Cerebrospinal fluid (CSF) is analyzed in the clinical pathology area rather than the anatomic pathology area.

B. Sputum fluid is analyzed in the clinical pathology area rather than the anatomic pathology area.

C. Synovial fluid is analyzed in the clinical pathology area rather than the anatomic pathology area.

D. In the anatomic pathology area, autopsies are performed and surgical biopsy tissues are analyzed. (p. 30)

47.

A. The encephalography section uses the electroencephalograph (EEG) to record brain wave patterns that will not be harmful to Ms. Pickins entering the area.

B. Ms. Pickins should avoid going to the radiotherapy section of the hospital, since the use of high-energy X-rays occurs in the treatment of disease such as cancer. Safety precautions are important to avoid unnecessary irradiation. (p. 31)

C. The physical therapy department will not be harmful to Ms. Pickins, since the department uses rehabilitation programs such as heat/cold, water therapy, and physical exercises for the patients.

D. The pharmacy department dispenses medications, and therefore Ms. Pickins should be safe if she needs to go to that department to pick up or drop off anything.

48.

A. Electrophoresis testing falls in the category of high-complexity test, since it is complex to perform and may allow for reasonable risk of harm to the patients if results are inaccurate.

B. Electrophoresis testing falls in the category of high-complexity test, since it is complex to perform and may allow for reasonable risk of harm to the patients if results are inaccurate.

C. Electrophoresis testing falls in the category of high-complexity test, since it is complex to perform and may allow for reasonable risk of harm to the patients if results are inaccurate. (p. 33)

D. Electrophoresis testing falls in the category of high-complexity test, since it is complex to perform and may allow for reasonable risk of harm to the patients if results are inaccurate.

49.

A. Primary health care is given to maintain and monitor normal health. It is also given to diagnose and treat colds or sore throats and to treat chronic illnesses such as diabetes mellitus. (p. 27)

B. Secondary care refers to specialized care in highly diagnostic and treatment services such as ophthalmology.

C. Tertiary care is highly specialized and oriented toward unusual and complex diagnoses and therapies. An invasive procedure such as open-heart surgery is an example of tertiary care.

D. Currently, there is not a level of health care called quarternary care.

50.

A. The clinical immunology/serology section performs testing procedures to detect various antibodies to diseases such as Legionnaire's disease antibody.

B. The clinical immunology/serology section performs testing procedures to detect various antibodies to diseases such as Legionnaire's disease antibody. (p. 35)

C. The clinical immunology/serology section performs testing procedures to detect various antibodies to diseases such as Legionnaire's disease antibody.

D. The clinical immunology/serology section performs testing procedures to detect various antibodies to diseases such as Legionnaire's disease antibody.

2 Basic Anatomy and Physiology of Organ Systems

chapter objectives

Upon completion of Chapter 2, the learner is responsible for the following:

➤ Describe the anatomic surface regions and cavities of the body.

➤ Identify the eight structural levels of the human body.

➤ Describe the role of homeostasis in normal body functioning.

➤ Describe the purpose, function, and structural components of the 11 body systems.

➤ Recognize examples of disorders associated with each organ system.

➤ List common diagnostic tests associated with each organ system.

DIRECTIONS Each of the questions or incomplete statements below is followed by four suggested answers or completions. Select **one answer** that is best in each case.

 KNOWLEDGE LEVEL = 2

1. Which of the following body systems provide carbon dioxide and oxygen exchange?
   A. nervous
   B. muscular
   C. respiratory
   D. reproductive

 KNOWLEDGE LEVEL = 1

2. Which of the following body systems is the primary regulator of hormones?
   A. digestive
   B. endocrine
   C. urinary
   D. integumentary

 KNOWLEDGE LEVEL = 1

3. The study of anatomy is best characterized by which of the following?
   A. functional components of the body
   B. biochemical makeup of the body
   C. structural components of the body
   D. anabolic and catabolic mechanisms in the body

 KNOWLEDGE LEVEL = 1

4. The pituitary gland is often referred to as:
   A. the respiratory control gland
   B. the "master gland"
   C. lymph tissue
   D. germ cells

 KNOWLEDGE LEVEL = 1

5. How many chromosomes are contained in human cells?
   A. 25
   B. 50
   C. 46
   D. 100

 KNOWLEDGE LEVEL = 1

6. What portion of human body weight is water?
   A. 90%
   B. half
   C. one-fourth
   D. two-thirds

 KNOWLEDGE LEVEL = 1

7. Meninges are defined as:
   A. causative agent of meningitis
   B. protective membrane layers
   C. control nerves
   D. control reflexes

 KNOWLEDGE LEVEL = 1

8. Which organ secretes bile?
   A. pancreas
   B. stomach
   C. appendix
   D. liver

KNOWLEDGE LEVEL = 1

9. Glomeruli are best described as:
   A. filters of the kidney
   B. cells in the liver
   C. part of the digestive system
   D. part of the endocrine system

 KNOWLEDGE LEVEL = 1

10. The endocrine system can best be evaluated by:
    A. tissue biopsy
    B. analyzing hormone levels
    C. doing blood gas analyses
    D. testing spinal fluid

 KNOWLEDGE LEVEL = 1

11. Physiology is the study of:
    A. functional components of the body
    B. mechanical makeup of the body
    C. structural components of the body
    D. anabolic and catabolic mechanisms in the body

 KNOWLEDGE LEVEL = 1

12. Which structure governs the functions of the individual cell such as growth, repair, reproduction, and metabolism?
    A. membrane
    B. cytoplasm
    C. lysosome
    D. nucleus

KNOWLEDGE LEVEL = 1

13. Cell metabolism involves energy production by:
    A. DNA transfer

B. perspiration
C. breaking down chemical substances
D. hemolysis

 KNOWLEDGE LEVEL = 1

14. Glycogen is best defined as:
    A. substance for aiding digestion
    B. hormone produced in the adrenals
    C. hormone used for cell division
    D. stored glucose in muscles

 KNOWLEDGE LEVEL = 1

15. How many lobes do normal human lungs have?
    A. 2
    B. 3
    C. 4
    D. 5

 KNOWLEDGE LEVEL = 1

16. How much air can a normal adult's lungs hold?
    A. about 1 quart
    B. about 3 to 4 quarts
    C. about 8 to 10 quarts
    D. about 15 quarts

 KNOWLEDGE LEVEL = 1

17. The molecule that transports oxygen and carbon dioxide is:
    A. alveoli
    B. chloride
    C. hemoglobin
    D. carbon

KNOWLEDGE LEVEL = 2

18. After oxygen crosses the respiratory membranes (in the lung) into the blood, about 97% of it combines with:
    A. the iron-containing heme portion of hemoglobin
    B. carbon dioxide
    C. hypochloride
    D. carbaminohemoglobin

 KNOWLEDGE LEVEL = 1

19. What is the pH range of a normal body?
    A. 0 to 7
    B. 6. 5 to 10
    C. 7. 35 to 7. 45
    D. 7. 5 to 8. 0

 KNOWLEDGE LEVEL = 2

20. As CO_2 levels increase in the blood, what happens to the blood pH?
    A. decreases
    B. increases
    C. stays the same
    D. increases for the first few minutes then drops to normal

 KNOWLEDGE LEVEL = 2

21. An XX pair of chromosomes means that the fetus will be:
    A. a baby boy
    B. a baby girl
    C. a brown-haired child
    D. a blue-eyed child

 KNOWLEDGE LEVEL = 1

22. Which of the following pairs are opposite regions or planes of the body?
    A. anterior/posterior
    B. distal/proximal
    C. lateral/medial
    D. all of the above

 KNOWLEDGE LEVEL = 2

23. The anterior or ventral surface of the body has which of the following body cavities?
    A. thoracic, abdominal, and pelvic
    B. abdominal only
    C. spinal
    D. cranial

 KNOWLEDGE LEVEL = 2

24. The posterior or dorsal surface is divided into which of the following cavities?
    A. thoracic, abdominal, and pelvic
    B. cranial and spinal
    C. abdominal only
    D. spinal only

 KNOWLEDGE LEVEL = 1

25. The posterior and anterior sections of the body are divided by which of the body planes?
    A. spinal
    B. ventral
    C. transverse
    D. frontal

KNOWLEDGE LEVEL = 1

26. Characteristics of the normal human body include:
    A. a backbone and organ cavities
    B. bisymmetry
    C. 11 organ systems
    D. all of the above

 KNOWLEDGE LEVEL = 1

27. The skeletal system:
    A. provides support, leverage, and movement
    B. secretes hormones
    C. provides pathways for nerve functions
    D. provides germ cell formation

 KNOWLEDGE LEVEL = 1

28. Homeostasis refers to:
    A. a chemical imbalance
    B. the steady-state condition
    C. an anabolism
    D. blood clotting

 KNOWLEDGE LEVEL = 1

29. Which of the following body systems provide protection and support and allow the body to move?
    A. integumentary
    B. skeletal
    C. nervous
    D. lymphatic

 KNOWLEDGE LEVEL = 1

30. Germ cells are defined as:
    A. energy producers
    B. neurons

C. sperm and ova
D. hair follicles

 KNOWLEDGE LEVEL = 1

31. The integumentary system consists of:
    A. skin and hair
    B. sweat and oil glands
    C. teeth and fingernails
    D. all of the above

 KNOWLEDGE LEVEL = 1

32. Functions of the skin include:
    A. prevention of water loss
    B. secretion of oils
    C. production of perspiration
    D. all of the above

 KNOWLEDGE LEVEL = 1

33. Which of the following body systems has the functions of communication, control, and integration?
    A. digestive
    B. integumentary
    C. nervous
    D. skeletal

 KNOWLEDGE LEVEL = 1

34. Melanin is described as:
    A. a pigment that provides skin color
    B. a covering for the brain and spinal cord
    C. a means of protecting tissues from infections
    D. a heat insulator

KNOWLEDGE LEVEL = 1

35. The sagittal plane of the body:
    A. divides the body into quadrants
    B. runs in a transverse plane
    C. divides the body into right and left halves
    D. divides the body into upper and lower sections

 KNOWLEDGE LEVEL = 1

36. DNA:
    A. is a double helix
    B. is located in the nucleus
    C. contains thousands of genes
    D. all of the above

 KNOWLEDGE LEVEL = 1

37. Bones and cartilage compose the skeletal system. They differ in some ways. Cartilage:
    A. allows for more flexibility
    B. is calcified
    C. is a very porous material
    D. is rigid

 KNOWLEDGE LEVEL = 1

38. Peristalsis is:
    A. a method of absorption
    B. a way to measure digestive capacity
    C. part of the stomach
    D. wavelike intestinal contractions that move food

 KNOWLEDGE LEVEL = 1

39. The skeletal system serves the body for:
    A. support and protection
    B. movement and leverage
    C. hematopoiesis and calcium storage
    D. all of the above

 KNOWLEDGE LEVEL = 2

40. Laboratory tests that evaluate the skeletal system include:
    A. serum calcium
    B. alkaline phosphatase
    C. synovial fluid analysis
    D. all of the above

 KNOWLEDGE LEVEL = 1

41. The nervous system is composed of:
    A. brain
    B. spinal fluid and spinal cord
    C. meninges
    D. all of the above

 KNOWLEDGE LEVEL = 1

42. Bones are categorized into which of the following groups?
    A. flexors
    B. ligaments
    C. joints
    D. none of the above

 KNOWLEDGE LEVEL = 2

43. Meningitis can be detected by:
    A. blood analyses
    B. urine cultures
    C. measuring carbon dioxide
    D. spinal fluid cultures

 KNOWLEDGE LEVEL = 1

44. Components of the respiratory system include:
    A. trachea and lungs
    B. intestine
    C. heart
    D. humerus

KNOWLEDGE LEVEL = 2

45. Laboratory testing of the muscular system would include:
    A. creatine kinase and lactate dehydrogenase
    B. synovial fluid
    C. urine culture
    D. serum calcium

KNOWLEDGE LEVEL = 1

46. Disorders of the skeletal system include:
    A. arthritis and bursitis
    B. gout
    C. bacterial infections
    D. all of the above

KNOWLEDGE LEVEL = 1

47. Muscles are classified into which of the following groups?
    A. skeletal or striated voluntary
    B. visceral or nonstriated (smooth) involuntary
    C. cardiac or striated involuntary
    D. all of the above

KNOWLEDGE LEVEL = 1

48. The nervous system is composed of:
    A. neurons, brain, and spinal cord
    B. blood cells and bone marrow
    C. cartilage coverings
    D. fluid

KNOWLEDGE LEVEL = 1

49. Sensory neurons:
    A. are cells that secrete adrenaline
    B. transmit nerve impulses to the spinal cord or brain

C. enable humans to respond in a sensible manner
D. cause emotional problems

KNOWLEDGE LEVEL = 1

50. Disorders of the nervous system include:
    A. encephalitis and meningitis
    B. Parkinson's disease
    C. amyotrophic lateral sclerosis
    D. all of the above

KNOWLEDGE LEVEL = 2

51. Respiration in the average person:
    A. allows for the exchange of cells
    B. occurs about 5 times per minute
    C. occurs approximately 20,000 times per day
    D. keeps the lungs soft and spongy

KNOWLEDGE LEVEL = 2

52. If a normal person breathes in, the O_2 travels through air passages to the lungs. Which of the following takes place?
    A. O_2 is exchanged for CO_2.
    B. The heart beats faster.
    C. The lungs can fill with fluid.
    D. The pulse rate changes.

KNOWLEDGE LEVEL = 2

53. Hyperventilation results when:
    A. you hold your nose
    B. the pharynx and larynx become contracted
    C. respiration becomes faster and deeper
    D. the lungs are releasing too much oxygen

KNOWLEDGE LEVEL = 1

54. The pharynx:
    A. releases hormones for respiration
    B. is a tubelike passageway for food and air
    C. begins to absorb oxygen as it passes through to the lungs
    D. all of the above

 KNOWLEDGE LEVEL = 1

55. Lungs:
    A. contain branches of alveoli with surrounding capillaries
    B. take in large amounts of oxygen
    C. release large amounts of carbon dioxide
    D. all of the above

 KNOWLEDGE LEVEL = 2

56. In lung capillaries, the partial pressure of carbon dioxide decreases and the partial pressure of oxygen increases. This causes:
    A. oxygen to combine with hemoglobin
    B. chemical combustion
    C. formation of free oxygen molecules
    D. hyperventilation

 KNOWLEDGE LEVEL = 1

57. The digestive system functions include:
    A. breaking down food and eliminating waste
    B. secreting hormones for regulatory functions
    C. transporting oxygen and carbon dioxide
    D. none of the above

 KNOWLEDGE LEVEL = 1

58. The GI tract includes the:
    A. mouth, pharynx, and esophagus

    B. stomach, intestines, gallbladder, and appendix
    C. salivary glands, teeth, and liver
    D. all of the above

 KNOWLEDGE LEVEL = 1

59. Disorders of the respiratory system include:
    A. ulcers
    B. pneumonia, influenza, emphysema, and cystic fibrosis
    C. melanoma
    D. none of the above

 KNOWLEDGE LEVEL = 1

60. The kidney's main function is to regulate:
    A. water
    B. electrolytes (sodium, potassium, chloride)
    C. nitrogenous waste products (urea)
    D. all of the above

 KNOWLEDGE LEVEL = 2

61. Metabolic acidosis occurs:
    A. in patients with diabetes mellitus
    B. when the body cannot eliminate adequate amounts of protein
    C. with a collapsed lung or blockage of respiratory passages
    D. all of the above

 KNOWLEDGE LEVEL = 1

62. STDs relate to:
    A. serotonin determinations
    B. hyperventilation episode
    C. collapsed lung
    D. none of the above

C. are located adjacent to the vocal cords

D. all of the above

63. Diagnostic tests for the endocrine system include:
    A. Pap smear
    B. ADH and ACTH levels
    C. occult blood
    D. cholesterol level

64. Metabolic acidosis results because of which of the following conditions?
    A. kidneys cannot eliminate acidic substances
    B. ingestion of vinegar
    C. excess elimination of hydrogen ions
    D. all of the above

65. Components of the lymphatic system include:
    A. lymph nodes
    B. tonsils
    C. bone marrow
    D. all of the above

66. Swollen lymph nodes:
    A. are common after infections
    B. are rarely detected by a physician
    C. can never be surgically removed
    D. are associated with varicose veins

67. Alveolar sacs:
    A. contain lymph nodes
    B. allow gas diffusion between air and blood

68. Bones consist of several layers. What is the inner layer of bone?
    A. compact bone
    B. synovial fluid
    C. cartilage
    D. spongy bone

69. Potassium hydroxide preparations are commonly used to diagnose:
    A. syphilis
    B. tuberculosis
    C. fungal infections on the skin
    D. none of the above

70. What component of bone produces most blood cells?
    A. compact portion
    B. marrow
    C. synovial fluid
    D. joints

71. Why does bone structure differ between males and females?
    A. Men have larger muscles.
    B. Women bear children.
    C. Blood vessels have different pathways in men and women.
    D. all of the above

FIGURE 2.1. Body planes.

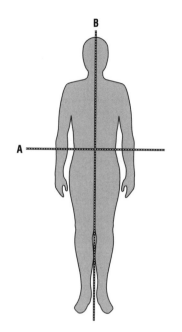
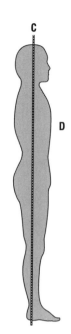

For Questions 72–75, refer to Figure 2.1 and match the body plane or region shown in the figure with the correct answer.

 KNOWLEDGE LEVEL = 1

72. The body region marked as "A" in Figure 2-1 represents which of the following?
    A. sagittal
    B. transverse
    C. dorsal/ventral
    D. cranial/caudal

 KNOWLEDGE LEVEL = 1

73. The body region marked as "B" in Figure 2-1 represents which of the following?
    A. sagittal
    B. transverse
    C. dorsal/ventral
    D. cranial/caudal

 KNOWLEDGE LEVEL = 1

74. The body region marked as "C" in Figure 2-1 represents which of the following?
    A. sagittal
    B. transverse
    C. ventral
    D. cranial

 KNOWLEDGE LEVEL = 1

75. The body region marked as "D" in Figure 2-1 represents which of the following?
    A. sagittal
    B. transverse
    C. ventral
    D. cranial

FIGURE 2.2. Diagram of venous drainage of abdomen and chest.

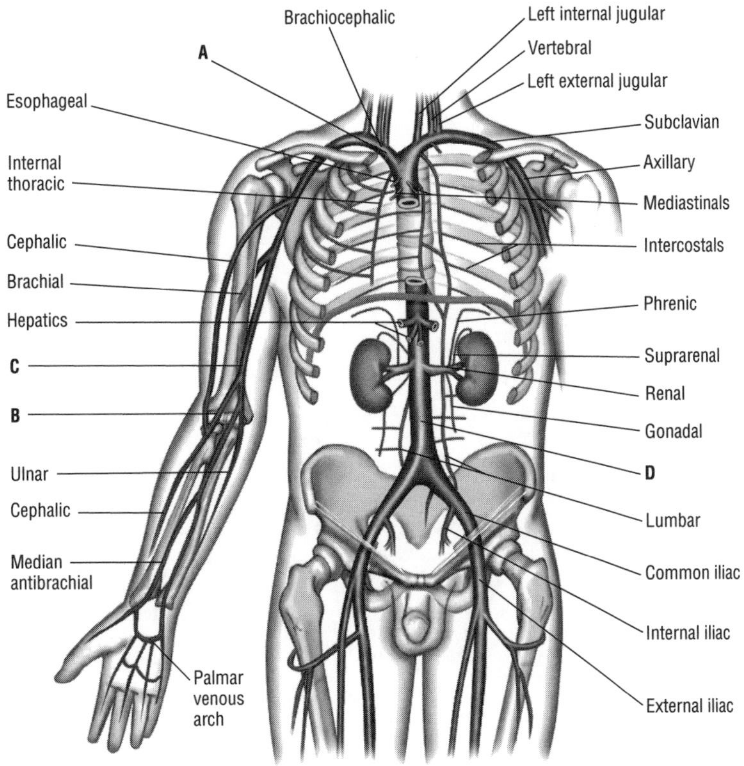

Labels in diagram:
Brachiocephalic
Left internal jugular
A
Vertebral
Left external jugular
Esophageal
Subclavian
Internal thoracic
Axillary
Mediastinals
Cephalic
Intercostals
Brachial
Hepatics
Phrenic
C
Suprarenal
B
Renal
Gonadal
Ulnar
D
Cephalic
Lumbar
Median antibrachial
Common iliac
Internal iliac
Palmar venous arch
External iliac

For Questions 76–79, match the labels on Figure 2.2 with the correct answers.

 KNOWLEDGE LEVEL = 1

76. The body region marked as "A" on the color plate represents the:
   A. inferior vena cava
   B. superior vena cava
   C. median cubital vein
   D. basilic vein

 KNOWLEDGE LEVEL = 1

77. The body region marked as "B" in Figure 2.2 represents the:
   A. inferior vena cava
   B. superior vena cava
   C. median cubital vein
   D. basilic vein

 KNOWLEDGE LEVEL = 1

78. The body region marked as "C" in Figure 2.2 represents the:
   A. inferior vena cava
   B. superior vena cava
   C. median cubital vein
   D. basilic vein

 KNOWLEDGE LEVEL = 1

79. The body region marked as "D" on the color plate represents the:
   A. inferior vena cava
   B. superior vena cava
   C. median cubital vein
   D. basilic vein

For Questions 80–83, refer to Figure 2.3 below and match the body plane or region shown in the figure with the correct answer.

 KNOWLEDGE LEVEL = 1

80. The vessel or region marked as "A" in Figure 2.3 represents the:
    A. alveolus
    B. capillary of the lung
    C. descending aorta
    D. aorta

 KNOWLEDGE LEVEL = 1

81. The vessel or region marked as "B" in Figure 2.3 represents the:
    A. alveolus
    B. capillary of the lung

    C. descending aorta
    D. aorta

 KNOWLEDGE LEVEL = 1

82. The vessel or region marked as "C" in Figure 2.3 represents the:
    A. alveolus
    B. capillary of the lung
    C. descending aorta
    D. aorta

 KNOWLEDGE LEVEL = 1

83. The vessel or region marked as "D" in Figure 2.3 represents the:
    A. alveolus
    B. capillary of the lung
    C. descending aorta
    D. aorta

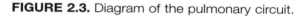

FIGURE 2.3. Diagram of the pulmonary circuit.

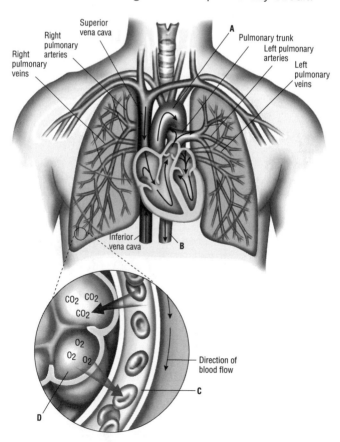

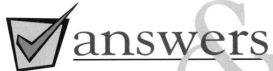

answers & rationales

1.

A. The nervous system is responsible for control and communication.

B. The muscular system is responsible for movement.

C. The respiratory system is involved in carbon dioxide and oxygen exchange. (p. 52)

D. The reproductive system is responsible for birth.

2.

A. The reproductive system is responsible for birth.

B. The endocrine system is the primary regulator of hormones. (p. 59)

C. The urinary system produces and eliminates urine.

D. The integumentary system is involved in the body's protection and regulation.

3.

A. Physiology is the study of functional components of the body.

B. Physiology includes the study of the body's biochemical make-up.

C. Anatomy is the study of structural components of the body. (p. 40)

D. Anabolic and catabolic mechanisms are reactions that produce energy and change complex substances into simpler ones, respectively.

4.

A. There is no such terminology as "respiratory control gland."

B. The pituitary is often referred to as the "master gland" because it controls and regulates many functions of the body through hormone production. (p. 59)

C. Lymph tissue is a vague term referring to the lymphatic system, which is responsible for maintaining fluid balance in the tissues, providing defense against disease, and absorbing fats from digestion.

D. Germ cells include ova and sperm.

5.

A. There are not 25 chromosomes in a normal human cell.

B. There are not 50 chromosomes in a normal human cell.

C. Normal human cells contain 46 chromosomes. (p. 58)

D. There are not 100 chromosomes in a normal human cell.

6.

A. The body is not 90 percent water.

B. The body is not half water.

C. The body is not one-fourth water.

D. Approximately two-thirds of the human body is composed of water. (p. 57)

7.

A. Meninges do not cause meningitis.

B. Meninges are the protective membranes that cover the brain and spinal cord. (p. 51)

C. Meninges do not control nerves.

D. Meninges do not control reflexes.

8.

A. The pancreas does not secrete bile; it manufactures and secretes insulin.

B. The stomach does not secrete bile; it secretes acid.

C. The appendix does not secrete bile or other substances.

D. The liver secretes bile. (p.56)

9.

A. Glomeruli are considered the filters of the kidney because they filter out water and solutes and reabsorb only the necessary amounts of these substances into the blood. Excess water and wastes are excreted as urine. (p. 56)

B. Cells in the liver secrete bile.

C. Glomeruli are part of the urinary system not the digestive system.

D. Glomeruli are part of the urinary system not the digestive system.

10.

A. Tissue biopsy would not reveal abnormalities in the endocrine system.

B. Since the endocrine system regulates hormone production, laboratory analysis of hormone levels is one way to evaluate abnormalities in this body system. (p. 59)

C. Blood gas analyses are useful for evaluating the respiratory system.

D. Spinal fluid analyses are useful for evaluating the nervous system.

11.

A. Physiology is the study of the functional components of the body. (p. 40)

B. Physiology is not the study of the mechanical make-up of the body.

C. Anatomy is the study of structural components of the body.

D. Anabolic and catabolic mechanisms are important in metabolism.

12.

A. The cell membrane is a protective barrier and allows substances to move in and out selectively.

B. The cytoplasm contains organelles and is composed mostly of water.

C. The lysosome releases digestive enzymes for food digestion.

D. The cell nucleus governs the functions of each individual cell. (p. 42)

13.

A. Metabolism does not involve DNA transfer.

B. Perspiration involves water loss from the skin.

C. Metabolism involves making necessary substances or breaking down chemical substances to use energy. (p. 45)

D. Hemolysis occurs when red blood cells rupture.

14.

A. Glycogen does not aid in digestion.

B. Glycogen is not a hormone produced in the adrenals

C. Glycogen is not a hormone used for cell division.

D. Glycogen is the form of stored glucose in muscles. Exercise increases the amount of glycogen available for muscles. (p. 50)

15.

A. Humans have 2 lungs with 5 lobes

B. Humans have 2 lungs with 5 lobes

C. Humans have 2 lungs with 5 lobes

D. Normal humans have two lungs. The left lung has only two lobes, and the right lung has three lobes. (p. 53)

16.

A. Normal lungs can hold more than 1 quart of air.

B. A normal adult's lungs can hold 3 to 4 quarts (approximately 3 to 4 liters) of air. (p. 53)

C. Normal lungs cannot hold 8 to 10 quarts of air.

D. Normal lungs cannot hold 15 quarts of air.

17.

A. Alveoli are grapelike structures in the lungs that allow diffusion of gases between air and blood.

B. Chloride is an electrolyte often evaluated in the laboratory.

C. Red blood cells transport O_2 and CO_2 as part of a molecule called hemoglobin. (p. 53)

D. Carbon is a building block of organic substances.

18.

A. Oxygen combines with hemoglobin in the capillaries of the lungs. (pp. 53–54)

B. Carbon dioxide does not combine with oxygen. It is exchanged for oxygen.

C. Hypochloride does not combine with oxygen.

D. Carbaminohemoglobin is a molecule containing hemoglobin and carbon dioxide.

19.

A. The normal human blood pH range is not 0–7.

B. The normal human blood pH range is not 6.5–10.

C. The pH of a normal human body has a narrow range of between 7.35 and 7.45. (p. 53)

D. The normal human blood pH range is not 7.5–8.0.

20.

A. As CO_2 levels increase in the blood, the blood pH decreases (becomes more acidic). As the CO_2 level in the blood increases, chemoreceptors in the brain cause a faster and deeper rate of respiration (hyperventilation) to blow off excess CO_2 from the body. (p. 54)

B. In this situation the pH does not increase.

C. In this situation the pH does not stay the same.

D. In this situation the pH does not increase for the first few minutes.

21.

A. In this situation the pH does not increase.

B. An XX pair of chromosomes indicates that the baby will be a girl. (p. 58)

C. In this situation the hair color cannot be determined.

D. In this situation the eye color cannot be determined.

22.

A. Anterior/posterior refer to opposite regions.

B. Distal/proximal refer to opposite regions.

C. Lateral/medial refer to opposite regions.

D. Opposite regions or planes of the body are anterior/posterior, distal/proximal, and lateral/medial. (pp. 40–41)

23.

A. The anterior or ventral surface of the body has the thoracic, abdominal, and pelvic cavities. (p. 40)

B. The anterior or ventral portions of the body contain other cavities in addition to the abdominal.

C. The spinal cavity is in the posterior or dorsal portion of the body.

D. The cranial cavity is in the posterior or dorsal portion of the body.

24.

A. The anterior or ventral surface contains the thoracic, abdominal, and pelvic cavities.

B. The posterior or dorsal surface is divided into cranial and spinal cavities. (p. 40)

C. The posterior or dorsal portions of the body contain other cavities in addition to the abdominal.

D. The posterior or dorsal portions of the body contain other cavities in addition to the spinal.

25.

A. "Spinal plane" is terminology that is not used.

B. The ventral surface of the body contains cranial and spinal cavities.

C. The transverse plane runs crosswise dividing the body into upper and lower sections.

D. The anterior and posterior sections are divided by the frontal plane, which runs lengthwise from side to side. (pp. 40–41)

26.

A. The human body has a backbone and organ cavities.

B. The human body is bisymmetrical.

C. The human body has 11 organ systems.

D. The human body has distinctive characteristics: a backbone, bisymmetry, body cavities, and 11 major organ systems. (p. 40)

27.

A. The skeletal system provides bodily support and allows for leverage and movement. (p. 48)

B. The endocrine system is primarily responsible for secreting hormones.

C. The nervous system provides pathways for nerve functions.

D. The reproductive system functions in germ cell formation.

28.

A. Chemical imbalance is the opposite of a steady state condition.

B. Homeostasis refers to a steady state or chemically balanced condition in the body. (p. 43)

C. Anabolism refers to energy production by cells.

D. Blood clotting is part of a process known as hemostasis.

29.

A. The integumentary system protects and regulates the body.

B. The skeletal system provides protection for internal organs and bodily support and allows for movement. (pp. 46–50)

C. The nervous system provides communication among body functions and intellectual processes.

D. The lymphatic system maintains tissue fluid balance and filters blood and lymph.

30.

A. Germ cells are not energy producers.

B. Neurons transmit nerve impulses.

C. Human sperm and ova are defined as germ cells. (p. 58)

D. Hair follicles are openings for hair to grow.

31.

A. The integumentary system includes skin and hair.

B. The integumentary system includes sweat and oil glands.

C. The integumentary system includes teeth and fingernails.

D. The integumentary system consists of skin, hair, sweat and oil glands, teeth, and fingernails. (pp. 46–47)

32.

A. Skin functions to prevent water loss.

B. Skin functions to secrete oils.

C. Skin functions to produce perspiration.

D. Skin prevents water loss and allows for perspiration as needed by the body during exercise, fever, or weather conditions. (pp. 46–47)

33.

A. The digestive system functions in the breakdown of food.

B. The integumentary system functions to regulate body temperature, receive sensory stimuli, and protect underlying tissues.

C. Both the endocrine and the nervous systems function for communication, control, and integration of bodily functions. (pp. 51, 59)

D. The skeletal system provides support and movement and produces blood cells.

34.

A. Melanin provides skin color and protects underlying tissues from absorbing ultraviolet rays from the sun. (pp. 46–47)

B. Meninges are coverings for the brain and spinal cord.

C. Melanin does not protect tissues from infections.

D. Melanin does not acts as a heat insulator.

35.

A. The sagittal plane does not divide the body into quadrants.

B. The transverse plane divides the body into upper and lower halves.

C. The sagittal plane runs lengthwise and divides the body into right and left halves. (pp. 40–41)

D. The transverse plane divides the body into upper and lower sections.

36.

A. DNA is a double helix.

B. DNA is located in the nucleus.

C. DNA contains thousands of genes.

D. DNA is described as a "double helix" or "twisted ladder." It is located in the nucleus and contains thousands of genes. It is not the same in all individuals, since it contains codes for the individual's genetic makeup. (p. 43)

37.

A. Cartilage is flexible and is surrounded by gelatinous material, in contrast to bone, which is calcified and rigid. (pp. 46–48)

B. Bone, not cartilage, is calcified.

C. Bone, not cartilage, is a very porous material.

D. Bone, not cartilage, is rigid.

38.

A. Peristalsis is not a method of absorption.

B. Peristalsis is not a way to measure digestive capacity.

C. Peristalsis is not a part of the stomach.

D. Peristalsis consists of wavelike intestinal contractions that aid the movement of food through the intestinal tract. (pp. 55–56)

39.

A. The skeletal system provides support and protection.

B. The skeletal system provides movement and leverage.

C. The skeletal system provides hematopoiesis and calcium storage.

D. The skeletal system provides bodily support, protection of internal organs, movement, leverage, hematopoiesis in the bone marrow, and calcium storage in bones. (pp. 47–48)

40.

A. Serum calcium is used to provide results for diagnostic and therapeutic monitoring.

B. Serum alkaline phosphatase is used to provide results for diagnostic and therapeutic monitoring.

C. Synovial fluid analysis is used to provide results for diagnostic and therapeutic monitoring.

D. Serum calcium, alkaline phosphatase, and synovial fluid analysis provide results for diagnostic and therapeutic monitoring. (p. 48)

41.

A. The brain is a part of the nervous system.

B. Spinal fluid and the spinal cord are part of the nervous system.

C. The meninges are a part of the nervous system.

D. The brain, spinal cord and fluid, and meninges are all functional components of the nervous system. (p. 51)

42.

A. Flexors is not a categorization of bones.

B. Ligaments are not part of bone structure.

C. Joints are not a category of bones.

D. None of the listed answers is appropriate. Bones are classified into four groups on the basis of their shapes. Long bones include leg bones and arm and hand bones. Short bones include wrist and ankle bones. Flat bones include several cranial bones, ribs, and shoulder blades. Irregular bones include some cranial bones and those of the vertebral column. (p. 48)

43.

A. Blood analyses alone cannot detect meningitis.

B. Urine cultures are not used to detect meningitis.

C. Measuring carbon dioxide is useful for evaluation of respiratory disorders.

D. Meningitis is detected by performing spinal fluid cultures. (p. 51)

44.

A. The nose, trachea, and lungs are all components of the respiratory system. (p. 52)

B. The intestine is part of the digestive system.

C. The heart is part of the cardiovascular system.

D. The humerus is a bone.

45.

A. Laboratory testing of the muscular system could include assays of specific muscle enzymes such as creatine kinase and lactate dehydrogenase, analysis of autoimmune antibodies, microscopic examination, or culturing muscle tissue biopsies. (p. 50)

B. Synovial fluid analysis would be useful in assessment of the joints.

C. Urine culture would be useful for diagnosing a urinary tract infection.

D. Serum calcium would be useful in assessing the skeletal system.

46.

A. Arthritis and bursitis are disorders of the skeletal system.

B. Gout is a disorder of the skeletal system.

C. Bacterial infections also affect the skeletal system.

D. Disorders of the skeletal system include inflammatory conditions (arthritis and bursitis); gout; bacterial infections such as osteomyelitis; porous bone conditions such as osteoporosis; developmental conditions such as giantism, dwarfism, and rickets; and bone tumors. (p. 48)

47.

A. Skeletal or striated voluntary muscles are attached to bones.

B. Visceral or nonstriated (smooth) involuntary muscles line the walls of internal structures.

C. Cardiac or striated involuntary muscles make up the heart wall.

D. Muscles are classified into (1) skeletal or striated voluntary, which are attached to bones; (2) visceral or nonstriated (smooth) involuntary, which line the walls of internal structures such as veins and arteries; and (3) cardiac or striated involuntary, which make up the wall of the heart. (p. 50)

48.

A. The nervous system is composed of specialized nerve cells (neurons), brain, spinal cord, brain and cord coverings, fluid, and the nerve impulse itself. (p. 51)

B. Blood cells and bone marrow are components of the cardiovascular system.

C. Cartilage is a component of the skeletal system.

D. The nervous system is not composed of fluid.

49.

A. Sensory neurons do not secrete adrenaline.

B. Sensory neurons (nerve cells) transmit impulses from muscle tissues to the brain or spinal cord. Motor neurons transmit impulses to muscles from the spinal cord or brain. (p. 51)

C. Sensory neurons are not responsible for sensible behavior.

D. Sensory neurons do not cause emotional problems.

50.

A. Encephalitis and meningitis are disorders of the nervous system.

B. Parkinson's disease is a disorder of the nervous system.

C. Amyotrophic lateral sclerosis is also a disorder of the nervous system.

D. Disorders of the nervous system include encephalitis, meningitis, tetanus, herpes, and poliomyelitis and conditions such as amyotrophic lateral sclerosis, multiple sclerosis, Parkinson's disease, cerebral palsy, tumors, epilepsy, hydrocephaly, neuralgia, and headaches. (p. 51)

51.

A. Respiration allows for the exchange of gases.

B. Inhalation occurs about 15 times per minute.

C. The average person inhales and exhales about 15 times per minute, or about 20,000 times per day. During the normal process of respiration, the exchange of carbon dioxide and oxygen takes place. (p. 52)

D. Inhalation does not keep the lungs soft and spongy; they are naturally spongy.

52.

A. As a person breathes, O_2 is exchanged for CO_2 in the lungs; the CO_2 is released when the person exhales. (p. 53)

B. The heart does not beat faster during normal respiration.

C. Lungs do not fill with fluid normally.

D. The pulse rate does not change during normal respiration.

53.

A. Holding your nose does not cause hyperventilation.

B. The pharynx and larynx do not become contracted during hyperventilation.

C. Hyperventilation results when the blood pH decreases while the CO_2 level in the blood increases. Chemoreceptors in the brain cause the body to breathe faster and deeper to blow off excess CO_2. (p. 54)

D. During hyperventilation, the lungs are not releasing too much oxygen.

54.

A. The pharynx does not release hormones for respiration.

B. The pharynx is a tubelike passageway that allows for the passage of food and air. Along with the larynx (voice box), it determines the quality of voice. (p. 52)

C. The pharynx does not absorb oxygen as it passes through to the lungs.

D. The answer did not include all of the above.

55.

A. Lungs contain branches of alveoli with surrounding capillaries.

B. Lungs take in large amounts of oxygen.

C. Lungs release large amounts of carbon dioxide.

D. Lungs contain branches of alveoli surrounded by capillaries. They are able to take in large amounts of oxygen and release carbon dioxide. They are soft and spongy and reach from just above the collarbone to the diaphragm. (p. 53)

56.

A. In lung capillaries, O_2 pressure [partial pressure of oxygen (PO_2)] increases and CO_2 pressure [partial pressure of carbon dioxide (PCO_2)] decreases, allowing O_2 to rapidly associate, or combine chemically, with hemoglobin and CO_2 to dissociate, or be released, from carbaminohemoglobin. Thus in the lungs, humans inhale oxygen and exhale carbon dioxide. (pp. 53–54)

B. Chemical combustion does not occur in the lung capillaries.

C. Oxygen molecules are quickly combined with hemoglobin in the lung capillaries.

D. Hyperventilation does not result in normal respiration.

57.

A. The digestive system functions, first, to break down food chemically and physically into nutrients that can be absorbed and used by body cells and, second, to eliminate the waste products of digestion. (p. 55)

B. The digestive system does not secrete hormones for regulatory functions.

C. The respiratory and circulatory systems transport oxygen and carbon dioxide.

D. "None of the above" is not an appropriate answer.

58.

A. The gastrointestinal (GI) tract includes the mouth, pharynx, and esophagus.

B. The gastrointestinal (GI) tract includes the stomach, intestines, gallbladder, and appendix.

C. The gastrointestinal (GI) tract includes the salivary glands, teeth, and liver.

D. The gastrointestinal (GI) tract includes the mouth, pharynx, esophagus, stomach, intestines, salivary glands, teeth, liver, gallbladder, pancreas, and appendix. (p. 55)

59.

A. An ulcer is a disorder of the digestive system.

B. Disorders of the respiratory system include tuberculosis, laryngitis, bronchitis, whooping cough, pneumonia, influenza, asthma, emphysema, cystic fibrosis, and tumors. (p. 52)

C. Melanoma is a type of skin cancer.

D. "None of the above" is not an appropriate answer.

60.

A. The kidneys regulate water in the body.

B. The kidneys regulate electrolytes (sodium, potassium, chloride).

C. The kidneys regulate nitrogenous waste products (urea).

D. The kidney's main function is to regulate the amount of water, electrolytes (sodium, potassium, chloride), and nitrogenous wastes in the body. (p. 56)

61.

A. Respiratory acidosis involves a drop in the pH of the blood below 7.35.

B. Respiratory acidosis results when the body cannot eliminate adequate amounts of CO_2.

C. Respiratory acidosis may result from a collapsed lung or blockage of respiratory passages.

D. Respiratory acidosis occurs during respiratory failure when the pH of the blood falls below 7.35, when the respiratory system is not able to eliminate adequate amounts of carbon dioxide in conditions such as collapsed lung or blockage of respiratory passages. (pp. 57, 52–55)

62.

A. Serotonin determinations are not useful or related to sexually transmitted diseases.

B. A hyperventilation episode is not related to sexually transmitted diseases.

C. A collapsed lung does not relate to sexually transmitted diseases.

D. STDs are sexually transmitted diseases. (p. 58)

63.

A. Pap smears are screening procedures for women to detect cancers of the reproductive system.

B. Diagnostic tests for the endocrine system include adrenocorticotropic hormone (ACTH) and antidiuretic hormone (ADH), among others. (p. 59)

C. Occult blood is used to detect blood in the stool.

D. A cholesterol level is used for assessing the predisposition to cardiovascular disease.

64.

A. Metabolic acidosis results because the body cannot eliminate acidic substances. (p. 57)

B. Metabolic acidosis does not result from the ingestion of vinegar.

C. Metabolic acidosis does not result from excess elimination of hydrogen ions.

D. "All of the above" is not an appropriate answer.

65.

A. Lymph nodes are only one component of the lymphatic system.

B. Tonsils are only one component of the lymphatic system.

C. Bone marrow is also a component of the lymphatic system.

D. The lymphatic system includes the lymph nodes, tonsils, bone marrow, spleen, and thymus gland. (p. 60)

66.

A. Swollen lymph nodes are common after infections. (p. 61)

B. Swollen lymph nodes are often detected by physicians.

C. Swollen lymph nodes are often surgically removed or cells are aspirated for analysis.

D. Swollen lymph nodes are not associated with varicose veins.

67.

A. Alveolar sacs do not contain lymph nodes.

B. Alveolar sacs are located in the lungs and allow diffusion of oxygen and carbon dioxide between air and blood. (p. 53)

C. Alveolar sacs are located in the lungs, not adjacent to the vocal cords.

D. "All of the above" is not an appropriate answer.

68.

A. Compact bone is the outer layer.

B. Synovial fluid is the lubricant between joints and bones.

C. Cartilage is similar to bone but it is surrounded by gelatinous material instead of a calcified substance.

D. The inner layer is the spongy bone or bone marrow. (p. 48)

69.

A. Syphilis is diagnosed using a blood test.

B. Tuberculosis is diagnosed by culture or acid fast staining techniques.

C. Potassium hydroxide (KOH) preparations are used to diagnose fungal infections of the skin. (p. 47)

D. "None of the above" is not an appropriate answer.

70.

A. Compact bone is the outer rigid layer of bone.

B. The bone marrow produces most blood cells. (p. 48)

C. Synovial fluid is the lubricant between joints and bones.

D. Joints allow for movement, they do not produce blood cells.

71.

A. Bone structure differs because of childbearing, not because of larger muscles.

B. Bone structure differs between men and women because the female pelvis is shallow and broad with a wider pubic arch to facilitate childbirth. (p. 48)

C. Bone structure does not differ between men and women because of different blood pathways.

D. "All of the above" is not an appropriate answer.

answers & rationales

For Questions 72–75, refer to Figure 2.1 to visualize the correct answers. Refer to the *Phlebotomy Handbook* for additional information.

72.

B. The body plane/region marked as "A" in Figure 2-1 represents the transverse plane, which runs crosswise or horizontally, dividing the body into upper and lower sections. (pp. 40–41)

73.

A. The body plane marked as "B" in Figure 2-1 represents the sagittal plane, which runs lengthwise from front to back, dividing the body into right and left halves. (pp. 40–41)

74.

D. The body region marked as "C" in Figure 2-1 represents the cranial (close to the head) or superior (above) region. (pp. 41–42)

75.

C. The body region marked as "D" in Figure 2-1 represents the ventral (front side) or anterior (in front of) surface of the body. (pp. 40–41)

FIGURE 2.1. Body planes.

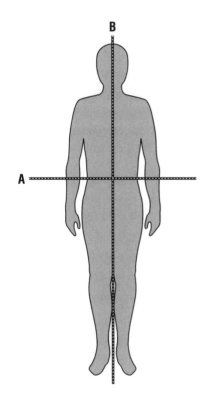
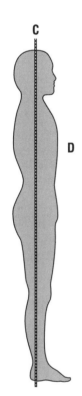

For Questions 76–79, refer to Figure 2.2 to visualize the correct answers. Refer to the *Phlebotomy Handbook* for additional information.

76.

B. The vein marked as "A" in Figure 2.2 represents the superior vena cava.

77.

C. The vein marked as "B" in Figure 2.2 represents the median cubital vein.

78.

D. The vein marked as "C" in Figure 2.2 represents the basilic vein.

79.

A. The vein marked as "D" in Figure 2.2 represents the superior vena cava.

FIGURE 2.2. Diagram of the venous drainage of abdomen and chest.

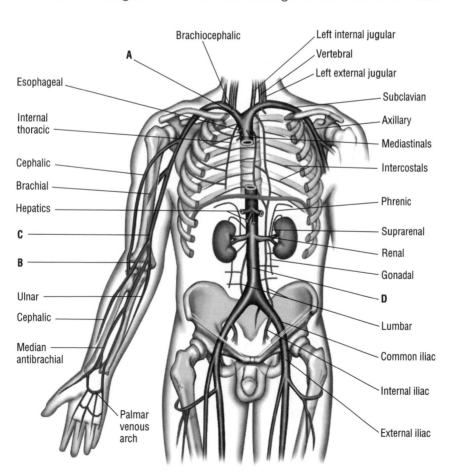

For Questions 80–83, refer to Figure 2.3 to visualize the correct answers. Refer to the *Phlebotomy Handbook* for additional information.

80.

D. The vessel or region marked as "A" in Figure 2.3 represents the aorta or aortic arch.

81.

C. The vessel or region marked as "B" in Figure 2.3 represents the descending aorta.

82.

B. The vessel or region marked as "C" in Figure 2.3 represents a lung capillary.

83.

A. The vessel or region marked as "D" in Figure 2.3 represents an alveolus of the lung, where oxygen and carbon dioxide exchange takes place.

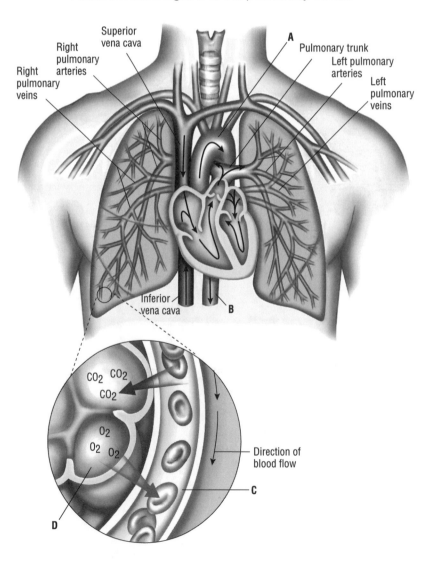

FIGURE 2.3. Diagram of the pulmonary circuit.

3 The Circulatory System

chapter objectives

Upon completion of Chapter 3, the learner is responsible for the following:

➤ Identify and describe the structures and functions of the heart.

➤ Trace the flow of blood through the cardiovascular system.

➤ Identify and describe the structures and functions of different types of blood vessels.

➤ Identify and describe the cellular and noncellular components of blood.

➤ Locate and name the veins most commonly used for phlebotomy procedures.

➤ Describe the phases of hemostasis.

➤ Describe how to take a person's blood pressure and pulse rate.

DIRECTIONS Each of the questions or incomplete statements below is followed by four suggested answers or completions. Select **one answer** that is best in each case.

 KNOWLEDGE LEVEL = 2

1. What happens to any region of the body that is deprived of blood for more than a few minutes?
   A. It dies.
   B. It shrinks.
   C. It makes the heart pump faster.
   D. It makes the person breathe harder.

 KNOWLEDGE LEVEL = 1

2. Another name for leukocytes is:
   A. red blood cells
   B. white blood cells
   C. platelets
   D. sera

 KNOWLEDGE LEVEL = 1

3. Another name for erythrocytes is:
   A. red blood cells
   B. white blood cells
   C. platelets
   D. sera

 KNOWLEDGE LEVEL = 1

4. Another name for thrombocytes is:
   A. red blood cells
   B. white blood cells
   C. platelets
   D. sera

 KNOWLEDGE LEVEL = 1

5. Serum is blood that:
   A. is highly oxygenated
   B. contains anticoagulant
   C. does not contain anticoagulant
   D. is rich in carbon monoxide

 KNOWLEDGE LEVEL = 2

6. Plasma is blood that:
   A. is highly oxygenated
   B. contains anticoagulant
   C. does not contain anticoagulant
   D. is rich in carbon monoxide

 KNOWLEDGE LEVEL = 1

7. Capillaries have which of the following characteristics?
   A. They carry deoxygenated blood toward the heart.
   B. They carry oxygenated blood away from the heart.
   C. They are microscopic vessels that link arterioles and venules.
   D. They carry only red blood cells.

 KNOWLEDGE LEVEL = 1

8. Arteries have which of the following characteristics?
   A. They carry deoxygenated blood toward the heart.
   B. They carry oxygenated blood away from the heart.

C. They are microscopic vessels that link arterioles and venules.

D. They carry only red blood cells.

 KNOWLEDGE LEVEL = 1

9. Veins have which of the following characteristics?

   A. They carry deoxygenated blood toward the heart.

   B. They carry oxygenated blood away from the heart.

   C. They are microscopic vessels that link arterioles and venules.

   D. They carry only red blood cells.

 KNOWLEDGE LEVEL = 1

10. Which of the following reflects the primary function of leukocytes?

    A. oxygen transport

    B. host cells

    C. blood clotting

    D. defense

 KNOWLEDGE LEVEL = 1

11. Which of the following reflects the primary function of erythrocytes?

    A. oxygen transport

    B. host cells

    C. blood clotting

    D. defense

KNOWLEDGE LEVEL = 1

12. Which of the following reflects the primary function of platelets?

    A. oxygen transport

    B. host cells

    C. blood clotting

    D. defense

 KNOWLEDGE LEVEL = 1

13. The process of blood cell development includes which of the following?

    A. They begin as undifferentiated stem cells.

    B. It occurs every 200 days.

    C. It occurs in the lungs.

    D. all of the above

 KNOWLEDGE LEVEL = 1

14. Which of the following features characterizes RBCs?

    A. biconcave disks that measure about 7 microns in diameter

    B. have no nuclei when circulating in the peripheral blood

    C. have a life span of about 120 days

    D. all of the above

 KNOWLEDGE LEVEL = 1

15. The blood vessels that carry oxygenated blood away from the heart are the:

    A. capillaries

    B. venules

    C. veins

    D. arteries

 KNOWLEDGE LEVEL = 1

16. The upper chambers of the heart are the:

    A. right and left atrium

    B. right and left ventricle

    C. inferior and superior vena cava

    D. none of the above

KNOWLEDGE LEVEL = 1

17. The chambers of the heart include the:
    A. right and left atria
    B. right ventricle
    C. left ventricle
    D. all of the above

 KNOWLEDGE LEVEL = 1

18. Which of the following statements describe(s) plasma?
    A. It contains clotted blood.
    B. It is normally bright yellow to orange.
    C. It is the fluid portion of unclotted blood.
    D. all of the above

 KNOWLEDGE LEVEL = 1

19. Which large artery or arteries carry blood to the body from the left side of the heart?
    A. venae cavae
    B. carotid
    C. mesenteric
    D. aorta

 KNOWLEDGE LEVEL = 1

20. Which of the following veins transports blood returning to the right side of the heart from the body?
    A. coronary vein
    B. portal
    C. inferior vena cava
    D. aorta

KNOWLEDGE LEVEL = 2

21. Which of the following answers describes the term "systole"?

    A. contraction of the heart
    B. relaxation of the heart
    C. blood tension
    D. a heart murmur

 KNOWLEDGE LEVEL = 2

22. Which of the following answers describes the term "diastole"?
    A. contraction of the heart
    B. relaxation of the heart
    C. blood tension
    D. a heart murmur

 KNOWLEDGE LEVEL = 1

23. The atrioventricular valves function to prevent:
    A. backward blood flow through the venae cavae
    B. blood flow from the atria to the ventricles
    C. blood flow from the ventricles to the atria
    D. backward blood flow from the aorta

 KNOWLEDGE LEVEL = 1

24. A "differential count" refers to:
    A. blood pressure
    B. contraction of the heart
    C. enumeration of specific types of WBCs
    D. a heart murmur

 KNOWLEDGE LEVEL = 1

25. Which arteries supply blood to the head and neck regions?
    A. hepatic
    B. subclavian
    C. brachial
    D. carotid

KNOWLEDGE LEVEL = 1

26. The hepatic artery delivers blood to the:
    A. liver
    B. heart
    C. legs and lower trunk
    D. arms

 KNOWLEDGE LEVEL = 1

27. Which arteries provide blood to the heart?
    A. hepatic
    B. subclavian
    C. coronary
    D. brachial

 KNOWLEDGE LEVEL = 1

28. Which of the following is the major artery in the antecubital area of the arm?
    A. brachial
    B. hepatic
    C. radial
    D. basilic

 KNOWLEDGE LEVEL = 1

29. Which of the following veins is most commonly used for venipuncture?
    A. median cubital
    B. femoral
    C. great saphenous
    D. brachial

 KNOWLEDGE LEVEL = 1

30. The term "buffy coat" refers to:
    A. erythrocytes and platelets
    B. leukocytes and platelets

C. mononuclear cells
D. protein and mineral deposits

 KNOWLEDGE LEVEL = 1

31. When blood exits the right ventricle, it travels via:
    A. the systemic circuit
    B. the pulmonary circuit
    C. the atrioventricular circuit
    D. none of the above

 KNOWLEDGE LEVEL = 1

32. How fast does the average adult heart beat?
    A. 50 to 55 times per minute
    B. 60 to 80 times per minute
    C. 90 to 100 times per minute
    D. 120 to 130 times per minute

 KNOWLEDGE LEVEL = 1

33. Which of the following instruments is used to measure blood pressure?
    A. a Coulter Counter (Coulter Electronics, Inc., Hialeah, FL)
    B. a pulse meter
    C. a differential counter
    D. a sphygmomanometer

 KNOWLEDGE LEVEL = 2

34. How is blood pressure reported?
    A. diastolic pressure alone
    B. systolic pressure alone
    C. diastolic pressure/systolic pressure
    D. systolic pressure/diastolic pressure

KNOWLEDGE LEVEL = 1

35. Universal donors are individuals with which blood type?
    A. A
    B. B
    C. AB
    D. O

 KNOWLEDGE LEVEL = 1

36. Which of the following best describes the term "hemostasis"?
    A. maintenance and retention of circulating blood in the vascular system
    B. vasoconstriction to prevent blood loss
    C. a steady-state condition
    D. clot retraction

 KNOWLEDGE LEVEL = 1

37. The term "fibrinolysis" refers to:
    A. clot retraction
    B. platelet degranulation
    C. vasoconstriction
    D. dissolution of clot and regeneration of vessel

 KNOWLEDGE LEVEL = 1

38. The term "intrinsic system" refers to coagulation factors contained in:
    A. tissues
    B. blood
    C. collagen fibers
    D. endothelial cells

 KNOWLEDGE LEVEL = 1

39. Tests for blood types and cross-match testing for donor blood are done in which of the following areas of the laboratory?

A. hematology
B. immunohematology
C. clinical chemistry
D. molecular pathology

 KNOWLEDGE LEVEL = 1

40. Which of the following represents a reference range for a platelet count?
    A. $50,000/mm^3$
    B. $50,000$ to $90,000/mm^3$
    C. $95,000$ to $100,000/mm^3$
    D. $250,000$ to $450,000/mm^3$

 KNOWLEDGE LEVEL = 1

41. Which of the following is a pressure point(s) used to check a patient's pulse?
    A. carotid artery
    B. brachial artery
    C. radial artery
    D. all of the above

 KNOWLEDGE LEVEL = 1

42. Which of the following statements best characterizes hemophilia?
    A. fear of needles
    B. fear of the sight of blood
    C. disease caused by internal blood clots
    D. excessive bleeding owing to inadequate clotting factors

 KNOWLEDGE LEVEL = 1

43. The longest vein in the body is the:
    A. greater saphenous
    B. median cubital
    C. aorta
    D. superior vena cava

KNOWLEDGE LEVEL = 1

44. Bone marrow samples are usually removed by:
    A. aortic puncture
    B. aspiration from the iliac crest of the hip
    C. heel puncture
    D. all of the above

 KNOWLEDGE LEVEL = 1

45. A reference range for RBCs would most likely be:
    A. 4.5 to 5.5 million/mm^3
    B. 10 to 20 million/mm^3
    C. 5,000 to 9,000/mm^3
    D. 1,000/mm^3

 KNOWLEDGE LEVEL = 1

46. A reference range for platelets would most likely be:
    A. 4.5 to 5.5 million/mm^3
    B. 10 to 20 million/mm^3
    C. 5,000 to 9,000/mm^3
    D. none of the above

 KNOWLEDGE LEVEL = 1

47. What are the clinical consequences if a patient is transfused with blood from a donor that has been misidentified or mistyped?
    A. Damage may result in the patient's kidneys.
    B. Damage may result in the patient's heart.
    C. It may result in death of the patient.
    D. all of the above

 KNOWLEDGE LEVEL = 1

48. Platelet functions are assessed in the laboratory using:
    A. anticoagulated venous blood
    B. coagulated venous blood
    C. bone marrow aspirates
    D. all of the above

 KNOWLEDGE LEVEL = 1

49. Hemoglobin content is assessed in the laboratory by analyzing:
    A. white blood cells
    B. erythrocytes
    C. megakaryocytes
    D. platelets

 KNOWLEDGE LEVEL = 1

50. Which of the following is the largest cell circulating in the peripheral bloodstream?
    A. erythrocyte
    B. megakaryocyte
    C. leukocyte
    D. platelet

For Questions 51–54, refer to Figure 3-1. The figure shows two blood specimens; the first tube contains an anticoagulant, and the second tube does not contain an anticoagulant.

 KNOWLEDGE LEVEL = 2

51. Which of the following answers corresponds to the label marked A?
    A. red blood cells
    B. white blood cells and platelets
    C. plasma
    D. serum

Figure 3.1. Blood specimens with and without anticoagulant, respectively.

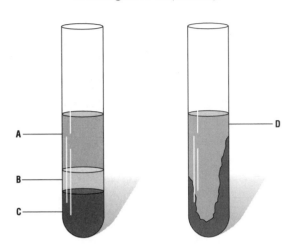

Figure 3.2. Major arm veins.

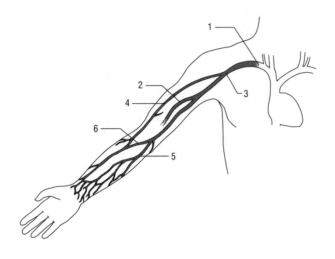

For Questions 55–60, refer to Figure 3-2.

KNOWLEDGE LEVEL = 2

52. Which of the following answers corresponds to the label marked B?
    A. red blood cells
    B. white blood cells and platelets
    C. plasma
    D. serum

KNOWLEDGE LEVEL = 2

55. The vein labeled 1 most closely resembles which of the following veins?
    A. subclavian
    B. axillary
    C. cephalic
    D. basilic

KNOWLEDGE LEVEL = 2

53. Which of the following answers corresponds to the label marked C?
    A. red blood cells
    B. white blood cells and platelets
    C. plasma
    D. serum

KNOWLEDGE LEVEL = 2

56. The vein labeled 2 most closely resembles which of the following veins?
    A. subclavian
    B. axillary
    C. cephalic
    D. brachial

KNOWLEDGE LEVEL = 2

54. Which of the following answers corresponds to the label marked D?
    A. red blood cells
    B. white blood cells and platelets
    C. plasma
    D. serum

KNOWLEDGE LEVEL = 2

57. The vein labeled 3 most closely resembles which of the following veins?
    A. subclavian
    B. axillary
    C. cephalic
    D. basilic

KNOWLEDGE LEVEL = 2

58. The vein labeled 4 most closely resembles which of the following veins?
    A. subclavian
    B. axillary
    C. cephalic
    D. basilic

 KNOWLEDGE LEVEL = 2

59. The vein labeled 5 most closely resembles which of the following veins?
    A. subclavian
    B. axillary
    C. cephalic
    D. basilic

 KNOWLEDGE LEVEL = 2

60. The vein labeled 6 most closely resembles which of the following veins?
    A. median cubital
    B. axillary

    C. cephalic
    D. basilic

For Questions 61–62, refer to Figure 3-3.

 KNOWLEDGE LEVEL = 2

61. Which of the following veins is the longest vein in the body?
    A. femoral
    B. greater saphenous
    C. popliteal
    D. lesser saphenous

 KNOWLEDGE LEVEL = 2

62. Which of the following veins comes up the lateral side of the ankle and goes deeper behind the knee?
    A. femoral
    B. greater saphenous
    C. popliteal
    D. lesser saphenous

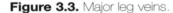

Figure 3.3. Major leg veins.

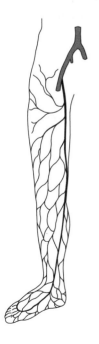
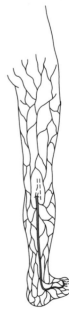

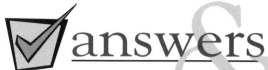
answers
& rationales

1.

A. Circulating blood provides nutrients, oxygen, chemical substances, and waste removal for each cell in the body. These functions are essential for homeostasis and life maintenance. Any region of the body that is deprived of blood may die within minutes. (p. 68)

B. Shrinkage of a body region is not one of the characteristics associated with deprivation of blood.

C. The heart will pump faster when the body is overexerting itself, as during periods of strenuous exercise or at high altitudes where there is less oxygen.

D. Respiration becomes faster and deeper also when the body is in situations in which it is overexerting such as during strenuous exercise.

2.

A. Erythrocytes are red blood cells.

B. Another name for leukocytes is white blood cells, or WBCs. White blood cells are divided further into cell lines that differ in color, size, shape, and nuclear formation. Leukocytes function primarily as part of the body's defense mechanism. (p. 71)

C. Platelets are thrombocytes.

D. Sera is the plural of serum, the fluid portion of coagulated blood. The other component of coagulated blood is composed of blood cells and coagulation factors that form the fibrin clot.

3.

A. Another name for erythrocytes is red blood cells, or RBCs. Approximately 99% of the circulating cells in the bloodstream are erythrocytes. They are biconcave disks that measure about 7 microns in diameter. Within each mature RBC are millions of hemoglobin molecules that function to carry oxygen to all parts of the body. (p. 69)

B. Leukocytes are white blood cells.

C. Platelets are thrombocytes.

D. Sera is the plural of serum, the fluid portion of coagulated blood. The other component of coagulated blood is composed of blood cells and coagulation factors that form the fibrin clot.

4.

A. Red blood cells are erythrocytes.

B. White blood cells are leukocytes.

C. Another name for thrombocytes is platelets. Platelets are much smaller than the other circulating cells in the bloodstream. Normally there are 250,000–450,0000 platelets/mm³. Platelets help in the clotting process by transporting needed chemicals to initiate the clotting process, slowing blood loss, and assisting in the formation of a clot. (pp. 69, 72)

D. Sera is the plural of serum, the fluid portion of coagulated blood. The other component of coagulated blood is composed of blood cells and coagulation factors that form the fibrin clot.

5.

A. In a normal blood specimen from a venipuncture, venous blood is not considered highly oxygenated.

B. If a blood specimen contains an anticoagulant, then a fibrin clot will not form and the specimen will be plasma.

C. Serum is the liquid portion of the blood that remains after a blood specimen has been allowed to clot. Blood cells remain meshed in a fibrin clot. (p. 73)

D. Carbon monoxide is a poisonous gas.

6.

A. In a normal blood specimen from a venipuncture, venous blood is not considered highly oxygenated.

B. Plasma is the liquid portion of a blood specimen that contains an anticoagulant. Anticoagulants are chemical substances that prevent blood from clotting. A blood sample that has been anticoagulated can be separated by centrifugation into plasma and blood cells. (p. 72)

C. If a blood specimen does not contain an anticoagulant, then a fibrin clot will form, and the specimen will be serum plus the blood clot.

D. Carbon monoxide is a poisonous gas.

7.

A. Veins carry deoxygenated blood toward the heart.

B. Arteries carry oxygenated blood away from the heart.

C. Capillaries are microscopic vessels that link arterioles to venules. They may be so small in diameter as to allow only one blood cell to pass through at any given time. Gas exchange occurs in the capillaries of tissues. (p. 77)

D. None of the blood vessels in the human body carry only red blood cells. All carry white blood cells, red blood cells, and platelets as well as other substances and chemicals necessary for sustaining life.

8.

A. Veins carry blood toward the heart (afferent vessels).

B. Arteries are highly oxygenated vessels that carry blood away from the heart (efferent vessels). They branch into smaller vessels called arterioles and into capillaries. They are normally bright red in color, have thicker elastic walls than veins do, and have a pulse. (p. 75)

C. Capillaries are microscopic vessels that link arterioles and venules.

D. None of the blood vessels in the human body carry only red blood cells. All carry white blood cells, red blood cells, and platelets as well as other substances and chemicals necessary for sustaining life.

9.

A. Veins carry blood toward the heart (afferent vessels). Because the blood in veins flows against gravity in many areas of the body, these vessels have one-way valves and rely on muscular action to move blood cells through the vessels. The valves also prevent back flow of blood. All veins except the pulmonary veins contain

deoxygenated blood, are dark red in color, and have thinner walls than arteries. The forearm veins that are most commonly used for venipuncture are the median cubital, basilic, and cephalic veins. (p. 77)

B. Arteries carry oxygenated blood away from the heart.

C. Capillaries are microscopic vessels that link arterioles and venules.

D. None of the blood vessels in the human body carry only red blood cells. All carry white blood cells, red blood cells, and platelets as well as other substances and chemicals necessary for sustaining life.

10.

A. Erythrocytes function primarily to transport oxygen to all parts of the body.

B. The term "host cell" does not apply to any blood cells.

C. Platelets function primarily as part of the blood clotting process.

D. Leukocytes function primarily as part of the body's defense mechanism. The cells phagocytize or ingest pathogenic microorganisms and play a role in immunity through antibody production. (p. 71)

11.

A. Erythrocytes function primarily to transport oxygen from the lungs to the tissues and carbon dioxide from the tissues to the lungs. (pp. 68–69)

B. The term "host cell" does not apply to any blood cells.

C. Platelets function primarily as part of the blood clotting process.

D. Leukocytes function primarily as a defense mechanism for the body.

12.

A. Erythrocytes function primarily to transport oxygen and carbon dioxide.

B. The term "host cell" does not apply to any blood cells.

C. Platelets function in the clotting process by transporting needed chemicals for clotting, forming a temporary patch or plug to slow blood loss, and contracting after the blood clot has formed. (p. 72)

D. Leukocytes function primarily as a defense mechanism for the body.

13.

A. Blood cells develop from undifferentiated stem cells in the hematopoietic or blood forming tissues such as the bone marrow. Stem cells are considered immature because they have not developed into their functional state. The cells will undergo changes in their nucleus and cytoplasm so that they differentiate and become functional once they are in the circulating blood. (p. 69)

B. The life span of each cell line differs: RBCs last about 120 days, WBCs last 1 day to several years, and platelets last 9-12 days.

C. Blood cell development does not occur in the lungs.

D. "All of the above" is not an appropriate answer.

14.

A. Red blood cells or erythrocytes measure about 7 microns in diameter, have no nuclei when circulating in the peripheral blood, and have a life span of about 120 days.

B. Red blood cells or erythrocytes measure about 7 microns in diameter, have no nuclei when circulating in the peripheral blood, and have a life span of about 120 days."

C. Red blood cells or erythrocytes measure about 7 microns in diameter, have no nuclei when circulating in the peripheral blood, and have a life span of about 120 days."

D. Red blood cells or erythrocytes measure about 7 microns in diameter, have no nuclei when circulating in the peripheral blood, and have a life span of about 120 days. (p. 69)

15.

A. Capillaries are microscopic vessels that link arterioles to venules.

B. Venules and veins carry deoxygenated blood toward the heart.

C. Venules and veins carry deoxygenated blood toward the heart.

D. Arteries carry oxygenated blood away from the heart. (p. 75)

16.

A. Upper chambers of the heart are the right and left atria. (Atlas Color Plate 1)

B. The right and left atria are the lower chambers of the heart.

C. The inferior and superior venae cavae are the largest veins in the body. The superior vena cava brings blood from the head, neck, arms, and chest; the inferior vena cava carries deoxygenated blood from the rest of the trunk and the legs.

D. "None of the above" is not an appropriate answer.

17.

A. There are four chambers in the human heart, which is located slightly left of the midline in the thoracic cavity. The upper chambers, or atria, are separated by the interatrial septum, and the interventricular septum divides the two ventricles, or lower chambers of the heart.

B. There are four chambers in the human heart, which is located slightly left of the midline in the thoracic cavity. The upper chambers, or atria, are separated by the interatrial septum, and the interventricular septum divides the two ventricles, or lower chambers of the heart.

C. There are four chambers in the human heart, which is located slightly left of the midline in the thoracic cavity. The upper chambers, or atria, are separated by the interatrial septum, and the interventricular septum divides the two ventricles, or lower chambers of the heart.

D. There are four chambers in the human heart, which is located slightly left of the midline in the thoracic cavity. The upper chambers, or atria, are separated by the interatrial septum, and the interventricular septum divides the two ventricles, or lower chambers of the heart. (p. 73)

18.

A. Plasma is from anticoagulated blood. It has not been allowed to form a clot.

B. Plasma is not bright yellow or orange.

C. The liquid portion of anticoagulated blood is called plasma. It is composed of 90% water and 10% solutes, which include nutrients, amino acids, fats, metabolic wastes, respiratory gases, regulatory substances, and protective substances. (p. 72)

D. "All of the above" is not an appropriate answer.

19.

A. The right side of the heart receives blood from the venae cavae.

B. The carotid artery is a large artery of the neck region.

C. The mesenteric artery is a large artery that feeds the intestines in the abdominal area.

D. When blood exits the left ventricle, it passes through the aortic semilunar valve and into the systemic circuit via the aorta. This circuit of vessels carries blood to the tissues of the body. (p. 74)

20.

A. The coronary veins serve the heart muscle itself.

B. The renal vein comes from the kidneys.

C. The inferior vena cava carries deoxygenated blood from the trunk and legs into the right atrium. (p. 74)

D. The aorta is the largest artery, not a vein.

21.

A. The heart's function is to pump sufficient amounts of blood to all cells of the body by contraction (systole) and relaxation (diastole). (p. 75)

B. Relaxation of the heart is referred to as diastole.

C. The term "blood tension" is not used.

D. A defective heart valve usually causes a heart murmur.

22.

A. Contraction of the heart is referred to as systole.

B. The heart's function is to pump sufficient amounts of blood to all cells of the body by contraction (systole) and relaxation (diastole). (p. 75)

C. The term "blood tension" is not used.

D. A defective heart valve usually causes a heart murmur.

23.

A. Atrioventricular valves are inside the heart, not in the veins outside the heart.

B. Normal blood flows through the heart from the atria to the ventricles.

C. The normal flow of blood in the heart goes from the atria to the ventricle. Atrioventricular valves prevent blood flow from going backward from the ventricle back into the atria. (p. 74)

D. Atrioventricular valves are inside the heart, not in the arteries outside the heart like the aorta.

24.

A. Blood pressure measurements are performed as part of a routine examination.

B. Contraction of the heart is referred to as "systole."

C. Results of a WBC differential count enumerate specific cell lines in percentages. (p. 83)

D. A heart murmur is usually caused by a defective heart valve.

25.

A. The hepatic artery serves the liver.

B. The subclavian arteries extend to the arms.

C. The brachial artery extends down the arm.

D. Right and left carotid arteries feed the head and neck regions. (Figure 3.2)

26.

A. The hepatic artery provides blood to the liver. (Figure 3.2)

B. The coronary arteries supply blood to the heart.

C. The femoral arteries supply blood to the legs.

D. The subclavian arteries supply blood to the arms.

27.

A. The hepatic artery supplies blood to the liver.

B. The subclavian arteries supply blood to the arms.

C. The coronary arteries supply blood for the heart muscle. (Figure 3.2)

D. The brachial arteries supply blood to the arms.

28.

A. The brachial artery is the major artery in the antecubital area of the arm. (Figure 3.2)

B. The hepatic artery serves the liver and is not located in the antecubital area of the arm.

C. The radial artery is in the lower part of the arm.

D. The basilic vein is located in the arm and does extend into the antecubital area.

29.

A. The median cubital vein serves as a connection between the cephalic and basilic veins. It is most commonly used for venipuncture because it is generally the largest in the area and is the best anchored vein in the area. (p. 77)

B. The femoral veins are in the leg.

C. The great saphenous veins are also in the legs.

D. The brachial vein is located on the upper arm and is usually a deeper vein.

30.

A. Erythrocytes settle below the buffy coat and platelets are part of the buffy coat.

B. The term "buffy coat" refers to the layer of white blood cells and platelets that form when plasma is centrifuged or if the cells are allowed to settle. It forms above the red blood cells and below the plasma. (pp. 72–73)

C. Mononuclear cells are only one type of cell within the buffy coat.

D. Protein and minerals are not found in the buffy coat.

31.

A. The systemic circuit carries blood to the tissues of the body.

B. When blood exits the right ventricle, it begins the pulmonary circuit, in which it enters the right and left pulmonary arteries. Arteries of the pulmonary circuit differ from those of the systemic circuit because they carry deoxygenated blood. Like veins, they are usually shown in blue on color-coded charts. These vessels branch into smaller arterioles and capillaries within the lungs, where gas exchange occurs (oxygen is picked up, and carbon dioxide is released). (p. 74)

C. The term "atrioventricular" refers to the valve between the atrium and the ventricle.

D. "None of the above" is an inappropriate answer.

32.

A. The average heart beats 60 to 80 times per minute, not 50 to 55 times.

B. The average heart beats 60 to 80 times per minute. Children have faster heart rates than adults do, and athletes have slower rates because more blood can be pumped with each beat. (p. 75)

C. The average heart does not beat 90 to 100 times per minute.

D. The average heart does not beat 120 to 130 times per minute.

33.

A. A Coulter Counter (Coulter Electronics, Inc., Hialeah, FL) is used to perform complete blood cell counts.

B. The term "pulse meter" is not appropriate.

C. A differential counter is used to count white blood cells.

D. A sphygmomanometer or blood pressure cuff is the instrument used to measure blood pressure. (p. 75)

34.

A. Blood pressure is not reported with diastolic pressure alone.

B. Blood pressure is not reported with systolic pressure alone.

C. Blood pressure is not reported as diastolic pressure/systolic pressure.

D. Blood pressure is reported as systolic pressure/diastolic pressure, such as 120/80. (p. 75)

35.

A. Type A donors are not universal donors because their red cells contain A antigen.

B. Type B donors are not universal donors because their red cells contain B antigen.

C. Type AB donors are not universal donors because they have both A and B antigens on their cells.

D. Individuals with blood type O are considered universal donors because their red blood cells can be transfused into a person with any ABO blood type. Their red blood cells do not contain A or B antigens to react with either Anti-A or Anti-B. (p. 71)

36.

A. Hemostasis is the maintenance of circulating blood in the liquid state and retention of blood in the vascular system by preventing blood loss. (p. 77)

B. Vasoconstriction to prevent blood loss is the first phase in the vascular process of minimizing blood loss. It is only one component of the hemostatic process.

C. A steady-state condition is known as homeostasis.

D. Clot retraction occurs when bleeding has stopped. It is the fourth phase in the hemostatic process.

37.

A. Clot retraction is phase four of the hemostatic process.

B. Platelet degranulation occurs during the second phase of the hemostatic process.

C. Vasoconstriction is the first phase in the vascular hemostatic process.

D. In the final phase of hemostasis, fibrinolysis occurs, whereby repair and regeneration of the injured vessel take place, and the clot slowly begins to dissolve as other cells carry out further repair. (p. 78)

38.

A. The extrinsic factors are stimulated when tissue damage occurs.

B. All coagulation factors required for the intrinsic system are contained in the blood. (p. 78)

C. Collagen fibers along with endothelial cells support the blood vessels; they do not have a direct impact on the clotting process.

D. Single layers of endothelial cells line the blood vessels and store some clotting factors.

39.

A. The hematology laboratory performs tests related to blood cells and coagulation indices.

B. Laboratory tests for blood typing and cross-matching for donor blood are performed in the immunohematology laboratory. (p. 83)

C. The clinical chemistry laboratory performs tests related to detection of chemical substances in the serum.

D. The molecular pathology laboratory performs a variety of tests on tissue or cells using tests that detect molecular abnormalities or utilize molecular probes.

40.

A. The reference range for platelets is 250,000 to 450,000/mm^3.

B. The reference range for platelets is 250,000 to 450,000/mm^3.

C. The reference range for platelets is 250,000 to 450,000/mm^3.

D. The reference range for platelets is 250,000 to 450,000/mm^3. (p. 69)

41.

A. When taking a pulse measurement, one begins by pressing two fingertips on an artery. The pulse is felt as a pressure against the fingertips. The best place to feel a pressure point is where the artery lies against a solid mass. The most common site is the radial artery of the wrist, at the base of the thumb. Other possible sites include the carotid, brachial, temporal, facial, femoral, popliteal, posterior tibial, and dorsalis pedis arteries.

B. When taking a pulse measurement, one begins by pressing two fingertips on an artery. The pulse is felt as a pressure against the fingertips. The best place to feel a pressure point is where the artery lies against a solid mass. The most common site is the radial artery of the wrist, at the base of the thumb. Other possible sites include the carotid, brachial, temporal, facial, femoral, popliteal, posterior tibial, and dorsalis pedis arteries.

C. When taking a pulse measurement, one begins by pressing two fingertips on an artery. The pulse is felt as a pressure against the fingertips. The best place to feel a pressure point is where the artery lies against a solid mass. The most common site is the radial artery of the wrist, at the base of the thumb. Other possible sites include the carotid, brachial, temporal, facial, femoral, popliteal, posterior tibial, and dorsalis pedis arteries.

D. When taking a pulse measurement, one begins by pressing two fingertips on an artery. The pulse is felt as a pressure against the fingertips. The best place to feel a pressure point is where the artery lies against a solid mass. The most common site is the radial artery of the wrist, at the base of the thumb. Other possible sites include the carotid, brachial, temporal, facial, femoral, popliteal, posterior tibial, and dorsalis pedis arteries. (pp. 76, 78)

42.

A. Fear of needles is not hemophilia; however, it is a common anxiety-producing feeling among patients before venipuncture.

B. Fear of the sight of blood is not hemophilia; however, it is a common anxiety-producing feeling among patients undergoing phlebotomy. Some individuals will faint at the sight of blood.

C. Overactive clotting can cause clots within the body, such as an embolus, thrombus, or disseminated intravascular coagulation disease.

D. Hemophilia is a disease that can cause excessive bleeding owing to abnormalities in the clotting factors. (p. 79)

43.

A. The greater saphenous vein is the longest in the body. It extends the length of the leg. (p. 80)

B. The median cubital vein is a vein of the arm.

C. The aorta is a large artery extending from the heart; it is not a vein.

D. The superior vena cava is a vein connecting to the heart. It brings blood from the head, neck, arms, and chest.

44.

A. Bone marrow cannot be aspirated from the aorta.

B. Bone marrow is aspirated from the iliac crest of the hip. A physician performs the aspiration. Marrow specimens can be stained and studied microscopically for the detection of abnormal numbers and morphological characteristics of blood cells. (p. 83)

C. Bone marrow cannot be aspirated from a heel puncture.

D. "All of the above" is not an appropriate answer.

45.

A. A reference range (sometimes referred to as the normal range) for a red blood cell count is 4.5 to 5.5 million/mm³. (p. 69)

B. Ten to twenty million cells/mm³ would be excessively high for a red cell count.

C. A count of 5,000 to 9,000 cells/mm³ is too low for a normal red cell count.

D. "None of the above" is an inappropriate answer.

46.

A. A reference range for a red cell count is 4.5 to 5.5 million/mm³.

B. A cell count of 10 to 20 million/mm³ is not a reference range for any blood cells.

C. A reference range for a white cell count is 5,000 to 9,000 cells/mm³.

D. None of the listed answers is appropriate. The reference range for a platelet count is 250,000 to 450,000 cells/mm³. (p. 69)

47.

A. All of the answers are correct. If a patient is transfused with blood that has been accidentally mistyped or confused with another patient's, the reaction can cause hemolysis of the cells in vivo, and/or RBCs can clump together, that is, agglutinate. This may result in damage to the kidneys, lungs, heart, or brain. The reaction can be fatal.

B. All of the answers are correct. If a patient is transfused with blood that has been accidentally mistyped or confused with another patient's, the reaction can cause hemolysis of the cells in vivo, and/or RBCs can clump together, that is, agglutinate. This may result in damage to the kidneys, lungs, heart, or brain. The reaction can be fatal.

C. All of the answers are correct. If a patient is transfused with blood that has been accidentally mistyped

or confused with another patient's, the reaction can cause hemolysis of the cells in vivo, and/or RBCs can clump together, that is, agglutinate. This may result in damage to the kidneys, lungs, heart, or brain. The reaction can be fatal.

D. All of the answers are correct. If a patient is transfused with blood that has been accidentally mistyped or confused with another patient's, the reaction can cause hemolysis of the cells in vivo, and/or RBCs can clump together, that is, agglutinate. This may result in damage to the kidneys, lungs, heart, or brain. The reaction can be fatal. (p. 70)

48.

A. Platelet function as well as each coagulation factor can be measured from anticoagulated blood specimens in the coagulation section of the clinical hematology laboratory. (p. 83)

B. Coagulated venous blood cannot be used to assess platelet function, since the clotting sequence utilizes the platelets.

C. Bone marrow aspirates cannot be used to assess platelet functions that occur in the peripheral blood. Platelets in the bone marrow are not fully mature and would function very differently.

D. "All of the above" is an inappropriate answer.

49.

A. White blood cells cannot be used to determine hemoglobin concentration because they do not contain hemoglobin.

B. Since hemoglobin is contained within the red blood cells, they must be lysed to release the hemoglobin for assessment. (p. 83)

C. Megakaryocytes cannot be used to determine hemoglobin concentration because they do not contain hemoglobin.

D. Platelets cannot be used to determine hemoglobin concentration because they do not contain hemoglobin.

50.

A. Erythrocytes have a cell size of 6–7 μm.

B. Megakaryocytes are large cells from which platelets derive. They are located in the bone marrow.

C. Leukocytes are the largest circulating blood cells with a size range of 9–16 μm. Megakaryocytes are larger cells from which platelets derive; however, they are located in the bone marrow. (p. 69)

D. Platelets are much smaller than other blood cells.

For Questions 51–54, refer to Figure 3-1. The figure shows two blood specimens; the first tube contains an anticoagulant and the second tube does not contain an anticoagulant.

51.

C. The label marked A corresponds to plasma. It contains fibrinogen and did not form a blood clot as did the second specimen. (pp. 72–73)

52.

B. The label marked B corresponds to the white blood cells and the platelets in the sample. (pp. 72–73)

53.

A. The label marked C corresponds to the red blood cells in the sample. (pp. 72–73)

54.

D. The label marked D corresponds to the serum, which resulted after the blood sample was allowed to form a clot. (pp. 72–73)

For Questions 55–60, refer to Figure 3-2 to visualize the veins on the diagram.

55.

A. The vein labeled 1 most closely resembles the subclavian vein. (p. 77)

56.

D. The vein labeled 2 most closely resembles the brachial vein. (p. 77)

57.

B. The vein labeled 3 most closely resembles the axillary vein. (p. 77)

58.

C. The vein labeled 4 most closely resembles the cephalic vein. (p. 77)

59.

D. The vein labeled 5 most closely resembles the basilic vein. (p. 77)

60.

A. The vein labeled 6 most closely resembles the median cubital vein. (p. 77)

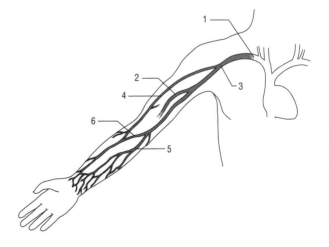

Figure 3.2. Major arm veins.

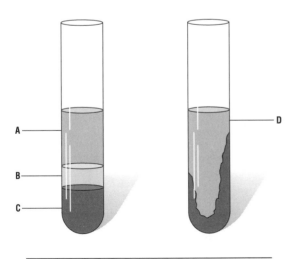

Figure 3.1. Blood specimens with and without anticoagulant, respectively.

Figure 3.3. Major leg veins.

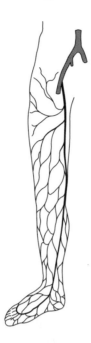
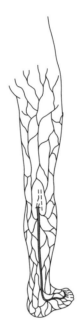

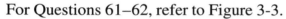

For Questions 61–62, refer to Figure 3-3.

61.

B. The greater saphenous veins are the longest veins in the body. (p. 80)

62.

D. The lesser saphenous veins come up the lateral side of the ankle and go deeper behind the knee. (p. 80)

SECTION II

Safety Procedures

4 Infection Control

chapter objectives

Upon completion of Chapter 4, the learner is responsible for the following:

➤ Define the term "nosocomial infection."

➤ Identify the basic programs for infection control.

➤ Explain the proper techniques for hand washing, gowning, gloving, masking, double bagging, and entering and exiting the various isolation areas.

➤ Identify the potential routes of infection and methods for preventing transmission of microorganisms through these routes.

➤ Describe the various isolation procedures and reasons for their use.

DIRECTIONS
Each of the questions or incomplete statements below is followed by four suggested answers or completions. Select **one answer** that is best in each case.

 KNOWLEDGE LEVEL = 3

1. Which of the following has the highest prevalence of nosocomial infections?
   A. urinary tract infections
   B. dermal infections
   C. respiratory tract infections
   D. wound infections

 KNOWLEDGE LEVEL = 1

2. Which of the following is *not* a component that makes up the chain of infection?
   A. mode of transmission
   B. source
   C. mode of transportation
   D. susceptible host

 KNOWLEDGE LEVEL = 2

3. Which of the following is considered a fomite?
   A. immunizations
   B. scrub suits
   C. transfusions
   D. hand washing

 KNOWLEDGE LEVEL = 3

4. Good nutrition can break the chain of nosocomial infections between the:
   A. source and susceptible host
   B. source and mode of transmission
   C. mode of transmission and susceptible host
   D. mode of transportation and susceptible host

 KNOWLEDGE LEVEL = 1

5. In Spanish, *peligro biologico* refers to the English term:
   A. hepatitis
   B. biohazardous
   C. blood-borne pathogen
   D. *Salmonella*

 KNOWLEDGE LEVEL = 2

6. Which type of isolation is frequently required for patients with infections that are transmitted by ingestion of a pathogen?
   A. respiratory isolation
   B. skin isolation
   C. enteric isolation
   D. reverse isolation

 KNOWLEDGE LEVEL = 2

7. Which of the following diseases usually require(s) strict, or complete, isolation?
   A. anthrax
   B. *Vibrio*
   C. *Shigella*
   D. *Salmonella* infection

 KNOWLEDGE LEVEL = 2

8. Which of the following interrupts the link between the susceptible host to the chain of infection?
   A. chemotherapy
   B. gene splicing
   C. radiation therapy
   D. good nutrition

KNOWLEDGE LEVEL = 1

9. The work status of a health care provider should be "off from work" if he or she has:
    A. gonorrhea
    B. hepatitis C
    C. herpes simplex
    D. chicken pox

KNOWLEDGE LEVEL = 2

10. Which of the following illnesses is usually transmitted from one person to another by coughing or sneezing?
    A. scabies
    B. Legionnaires' disease
    C. impetigo
    D. weeping dermatitis

KNOWLEDGE LEVEL = 2

11. Vectors in transmitting infectious diseases include:
    A. age
    B. mites
    C. rabies
    D. *Salmonella*

KNOWLEDGE LEVEL = 3

12. Babies whose mothers have which of the following problems must be isolated from other infants?
    A. cancer
    B. genital herpes
    C. kidney failure and are in a dialysis unit
    D. burns

KNOWLEDGE LEVEL = 2

13. A nosocomial infection occurs when:
    A. a source is detected
    B. the chain of infection is complete
    C. a means of transmission is maintained by disinfectants
    D. a susceptible host remains stable

KNOWLEDGE LEVEL = 1

14. Disinfectants are:
    A. chemicals that are used to inhibit the growth and development of microorganisms but do not necessarily kill them
    B. used frequently on skin
    C. chemicals that are used to remove or kill pathogenic microorganisms
    D. quaternary ammonium compounds

KNOWLEDGE LEVEL = 3

15. Which of the following is a commonly occurring pathogenic agent that causes nosocomial infections of the gastrointestinal tract?
    A. *Neisseria gonorrhoeae*
    B. *Vibrio cholerae*
    C. *Haemophilus vaginalis*
    D. *Bordetella pertussis*

KNOWLEDGE LEVEL = 2

16. Which of the following nosocomial infections usually has a 40 percent prevalence rate?
    A. bacteremia
    B. wound infections
    C. respiratory infections
    D. urinary tract infections

KNOWLEDGE LEVEL = 2

17. Which of the following chemical compounds is an antiseptic for skin?
    A. 1 percent phenol
    B. hexachlorophene
    C. chlorophenol
    D. ethylene oxide

 KNOWLEDGE LEVEL = 2

18. A commonly identified causative agent of nosocomial infections in the nursery unit is:
    A. *Escherichia coli*
    B. *Haemophilus vaginalis*
    C. *Shigella*
    D. *Vibrio cholerae*

 KNOWLEDGE LEVEL = 1

19. Reverse isolation is commonly used for patients who have:
    A. *Vibrio cholerae*
    B. immunodeficiency disorders
    C. hepatitis A
    D. whooping cough

 KNOWLEDGE LEVEL = 2

20. Which of the following is a commonly identified pathogenic microorganism that causes nosocomial skin infections?
    A. *Candida albicans*
    B. *Haemophilus influenzae*
    C. *Haemophilus vaginalis*
    D. *Moraxella lacunata*

 KNOWLEDGE LEVEL = 1

21. Antiseptics for skin include:
    A. hypochlorite solution
    B. formaldehyde

C. iodine
D. ethylene oxide

 KNOWLEDGE LEVEL = 1

22. Which of the following chemicals should be used to disinfect tourniquets and items contaminated with blood?
    A. 70 percent isopropyl
    B. 1:10 dilution of chlorine bleach
    C. hydrogen peroxide
    D. iodophors

 KNOWLEDGE LEVEL = 1

23. Which of the following types of nosocomial infections are most prevalent?
    A. dermal infections
    B. wound infections
    C. respiratory infections
    D. urinary tract infections

 KNOWLEDGE LEVEL = 2

24. Under the new CDC isolation guidelines, the old categories of isolation and disease-specific precautions have been collapsed into three sets of precautions that include:
    A. airborne, droplet, and contact
    B. airborne, respiratory, and contact
    C. enteric, contact, and respiratory
    D. complete, droplet, and airborne

 KNOWLEDGE LEVEL = 3

25. Using the new CDC isolation guidelines, standard precautions are a combination of the:
    A. complete isolation technique and body substance isolation
    B. universal precautions and body substance isolation
    C. enteric isolation technique, universal precautions, and complete isolation technique

D. contact isolation technique, complete isolation technique, and tuberculosis isolation

KNOWLEDGE LEVEL = 2

26. Which of the following isolation techniques requires that any blood collection equipment taken into the patient's room must be taken out after the blood is collected?
    A. enteric isolation
    B. respiratory isolation
    C. contact isolation
    D. reverse isolation

KNOWLEDGE LEVEL = 1

27. The following isolation technique is sometimes referred to as AFB isolation:
    A. body substance isolation
    B. tuberculosis isolation
    C. enteric isolation
    D. contact isolation

KNOWLEDGE LEVEL = 2

28. A factor that increases a host's susceptibility in the chain of infection is:
    A. drug use
    B. an immunization
    C. use of disposable equipment
    D. proper nutrition

KNOWLEDGE LEVEL = 3

29. Contact isolation may be required for patients infected with:
    A. infectious tuberculosis
    B. antibiotic-resistant microorganisms
    C. *Salmonella*
    D. *Shigella*

KNOWLEDGE LEVEL = 3

30. A phlebotomist had to avoid contact with patients for 24 hours after being started on an appropriate antibiotic and appearing symptom free. What type of infection could he or she have acquired for the above work limitations to apply?
    A. rubella
    B. chickenpox
    C. measles
    D. strep throat (group A)

KNOWLEDGE LEVEL = 2

31. In health care facilities, which is a typical fomite?
    A. phlebotomy tray
    B. 70% isopropyl alcohol
    C. hexachlorophene
    D. iodine for blood culture collections

KNOWLEDGE LEVEL = 2

32. In the process of preparing to enter a patient's room in isolation, which of the following would occur first?
    A. donning gloves and positioning them
    B. untying gown at the neck
    C. discarding mask
    D. donning mask

KNOWLEDGE LEVEL = 1

33. Which of the following is the most important procedure in the prevention of disease transmission in health care institutions?
    A. use of personal protection equipment
    B. use of appropriate waste disposal practices
    C. hand washing
    D. reporting personal illnesses to supervisor

KNOWLEDGE LEVEL = 2

34. Which of the following would require respiratory isolation?
    A. *Campylobacter* infection
    B. *Vibrio*
    C. mumps
    D. *Clostridium difficile*

 KNOWLEDGE LEVEL = 3

35. Which of the following is designed to reduce the risk of transmission of microorganisms from both recognized and unrecognized sources of infection in health care facilities?
    A. drainage/secretion isolation
    B. enteric isolation
    C. complete isolation
    D. standard precautions

 KNOWLEDGE LEVEL = 1

36. Which of the following organizations requires the development and implementation of an infection control program in a health care facility?
    A. JCAHO
    B. ASCP
    C. CLIA
    D. CLT

 KNOWLEDGE LEVEL = 2

37. The classification of infections according to prevalence rates is referred to as:
    A. infection control surveillance
    B. a nosocomial infection
    C. an employee health monitoring program
    D. chain of infection

 KNOWLEDGE LEVEL = 1

38. The following agency of the U.S. Department of Labor requires employers to provide measures that will protect workers exposed to biological hazards:
    A. JCAHO
    B. FDA
    C. OSHA
    D. NCCLS

 KNOWLEDGE LEVEL = 1

39. BSI in infection control protocol refers to:
    A. blood substance isolation
    B. blood serum isolation
    C. body substance isolation
    D. body sputum isolation

 KNOWLEDGE LEVEL = 2

40. Which of the following laboratory-acquired infections is most prevalent?
    A. HIV infection
    B. Rocky Mountain spotted fever
    C. hepatitis A infection
    D. amebic dysentery

 KNOWLEDGE LEVEL 1

41. If an accident occurs, such as a needlestick, the injured health care provider should immediately:
    A. contact his or her immediate supervisor
    B. fill out the necessary health care forms
    C. cleanse the area with isopropyl alcohol and apply an adhesive bandage
    D. take the needle back to the clinical laboratory for verification of the accident

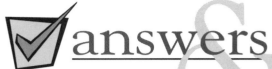
answers & rationales

1.

A. The highest prevalence of nosocomial infections occurs in urinary tract infections with a 40 percent prevalence rate. (p. 95)

B. The dermal infections prevalence rate for nosocomial infections is only 5 percent compared to the urinary tract infection prevalence rate of 40 percent.

C. The respiratory tract infection prevalence rate for nosocomial infections is only 15 percent compared to the urinary tract infection prevalence rate of 40 percent.

D. The wound infection prevalence rate for nosocomial infections is only 25 percent compared to the urinary tract infection prevalence rate of 40 percent.

2.

A. The three components that make up the chain are the source, mode of transmission, and susceptible host.

B. The three components that make up the chain are the source, mode of transmission, and susceptible host.

C. The three components that make up the chain are the source, mode of transmission, and susceptible host. (p. 101)

D. The three components that make up the chain are the source, mode of transmission, and susceptible host.

3.

A. Immunizations interrupt the infectious process. Scrub suits, computer keyboards, doorknobs, and telephones are a few examples of fomites.

B. Scrub suits, computer keyboards, doorknobs, and telephones are a few examples of fomites (objects that can harbor infectious agents and transmit infections). (p. 100)

C. Transfusions are given to interrupt the chain of nosocomial infections and are not fomites. Scrub suits, computer keyboards, doorknobs, and telephones are a few examples of fomites.

D. Hand washing is performed to interrupt the infectious process of nosocomial infections and therefore is not a fomite. Scrub suits, computer keyboards, doorknobs, and telephones are a few examples of fomites.

4.

A. Good nutrition is an important factor in interrupting the chain of nosocomial infections between the source and susceptible host. (p. 101)

B. Good nutrition is an important factor in interrupting the chain of nosocomial infections between the source and susceptible host.

C. Good nutrition is an important factor in interrupting the chain of nosocomial infections between the source and susceptible host.

D. Good nutrition is an important factor in interrupting the chain of nosocomial infections between the source and susceptible host.

5.

A. In Spanish, *peligro biologico* refers to the English term "biohazardous."

B. In Spanish, *peligro biologico* refers to the English term "biohazardous." (p. 109)

C. In Spanish, *peligro biologico* refers to the English term "biohazardous."

D. In Spanish, *peligro biologico* refers to the English term "biohazardous."

6.

A. Respiratory isolation has been required for patients with infections that may be transmitted over short distances through the air.

B. Skin isolation is not a type of isolation.

C. Enteric isolation is frequently required for patients with infections that are transmitted by ingestion of a pathogen. (p. 104)

D. Patients are put in reverse isolation not because they have an infection, but because they are highly susceptible to infection and need to be protected from the external environment.

7.

A. Strict, or complete, isolation is required for patients with contagious diseases that may be transmitted by direct contact or by air. For example, patients with anthrax require strict, or complete, isolation. (p. 102)

B. A person with a *Vibrio* infection would be placed in enteric isolation.

C. A person with a *Shigella* infection would be placed in enteric isolation.

D. A person with a *Salmonella* infection would be placed in enteric isolation.

8.

A. Chemotherapy is an agent that interrupts growth of cancerous cells but is not considered a factor in the chain of nosocomial infection.

B. Gene splicing is a new treatment involving DNA resynthesis in the patient. However, it is not used to interrupt the chain of nosocomial infection.

C. Radiation therapy is a treatment to destroy cancerous growths in patients but is not considered a factor in the chain of nosocomial infections.

D. Good nutrition interrupts the chain of nosocomial infection between the susceptible host and the source. (p. 101)

9.

A. An employee having gonorrhea may work.

B. An employee who has hepatitis C may work as long as his or her blood or body fluids are not exposed to anyone else.

C. An employee who has herpes simplex may work.

D. For seven days after eruption of chicken pox, the employee should not work. (p. 97)

10.

A. Scabies is a skin infection caused by mites, not by microscopic airborne droplets.

B. Legionnaires' disease is transmitted by microscopic airborne droplets. (p. 99)

C. Impetigo is a systemic infection caused by *Staphylococcus* and is transmitted through direct contact, not airborne droplets.

D. Weeping dermatitis is a skin disorder usually caused by an allergic response (i.e., wearing gloves).

11.

A. Age is not a vector. Vectors are insects and rodents that carry and transmit infectious diseases.

B. Mites act as vectors in transmitting infectious diseases. (p. 100)

C. Rabies is a disease caused by a virus, whereas a vector is an insect or rodent that carries and transmits infectious diseases.

D. *Salmonella* is a type of bacteria, not a vector.

12.

A. Babies whose mothers have genital herpes must be isolated from other infants.

B. Babies whose mothers have genital herpes must be isolated from other infants. (p. 110)

C. Babies whose mothers have genital herpes must be isolated from other infants.

D. A baby whose mother has been burned is not isolated, but the mother may have to be isolated to protect her from obtaining an infection.

13.

A. Nosocomial infections occur when the chain of infection is complete. The three components that make up the chain are source, mode of transmission, and susceptible host.

B. Nosocomial infections occur when the chain of infection is complete. The three components that make up the chain are the source, mode of transmission, and susceptible host. (pp. 100–101)

C. Nosocomial infections occur when the chain of infection is complete. The three components that make up the chain are source, mode of transmission, and susceptible host.

D. Nosocomial infections occur when the chain of infection is complete. The three components that make up the chain are source, mode of transmission, and susceptible host.

14.

A. Antiseptics are chemicals that are used to inhibit the growth and development of microorganisms but do not necessarily kill them.

B. Disinfectants are strong chemicals and are not used frequently on skin.

C. Disinfectants are chemical compounds that are used to remove or kill pathogenic microorganisms. (p. 118)

D. Quaternary ammonium compounds are antiseptics for skin that are found in many soaps.

15.

A. *Neisseria gonorrhoeae* is a pathogenic agent that causes nosocomial infections in the genital tract.

B. *Vibrio cholerae* is a pathogenic agent that causes nosocomial infections of the gastrointestinal tract. (p. 96)

C. *Haemophilus vaginalis* is a microorganism that causes nosocomial infections in the genital tract.

D. *Bordetella pertussis* is a bacteria that causes nosocomial infections in the respiratory tract.

16.

A. Bacteremia has a 5 percent prevalence rate of nosocomial infections.

B. Wound infections have a 25 percent prevalence rate of nosocomial infections.

C. Respiratory infections have a 15 percent prevalence rate of nosocomial infections.

D. Urinary tract infections have a 40 percent prevalence rate of nosocomial infections. (p. 95)

17.

A. 1 percent phenol is a disinfectant and is not used on skin.

B. Hexachlorophene is an antiseptic for skin that is used frequently in surgery. (p. 118)

C. Chlorophenol is a disinfectant and toxic for skin use.

D. Ethylene oxide is a disinfectant and toxic for skin use.

18.

A. *Escherichia coli* is a commonly identified pathogenic agent that causes nosocomial infections in the nursery unit. (p. 96)

B. *Haemophilus vaginalis* is a commonly identified pathogenic microorganism that causes nosocomial infections in the genital tract.

C. *Shigella* is a commonly identified pathogenic microorganism that causes nosocomial infections in the gastrointestinal tract.

D. *Vibrio cholerae* is a commonly identified pathogenic microorganism that causes nosocomial infections in the gastrointestinal tract.

19.

A. Enteric isolation is used for patients with infections that are transmitted by ingestion of the pathogen causing diarrheal diseases such as *Vibrio cholerae*.

B. Reverse, or protective, isolation is used for patients who have immunodeficiency disorders to protect them from the external environments. (p. 110)

C. Enteric isolation is used for patients with infections that are transmitted by ingestion of the pathogen causing diarrheal diseases such as hepatitis A.

D. Respiratory isolation is required for patients with infections that may be transmitted by air droplets such as in whooping cough.

20.

A. *Candida albicans* is a commonly identified pathogenic agent that causes nosocomial skin infections. (p. 96)

B. *Haemophilus influenzae* is a pathogenic microorganism that causes nosocomial ear infections.

C. *Haemophilus vaginalis* is a pathogenic microorganism that causes genital tract infections.

D. *Moraxella lacunata* is a commonly identified pathogenic agent that causes nosocomial eye infections.

21.

A. Hypochlorite solutions are disinfectants used on surfaces and instruments for cleansing but not skin because of their corrosive effects to skin.

B. Formaldehyde is a disinfectant having noxious fumes.

C. Iodine solutions are commonly used to cleanse the skin for blood culture collections. (p. 118)

D. Ethylene oxide is a disinfectant that is toxic and corrosive for cleansing the skin.

22.

A. A disinfectant having a chlorine bleach dilution of 1:10 or a disinfectant with a product label stating that it is HIV-cidal or tuberculocidal should be used to disinfect tourniquets and items contaminated with blood or other body fluids.

B. A disinfectant having a chlorine bleach dilution of 1:10 or a disinfectant with a product label stating that it is HIV-cidal or tuberculocidal should be used to disinfect tourniquets and items contaminated with blood or other body fluids. (p. 110)

C. A disinfectant having a chlorine bleach dilution of 1:10 or a disinfectant with a product label stating that it is HIV-cidal or tuberculocidal should be used to disinfect tourniquets and items contaminated with blood or other body fluids.

D. A disinfectant having a chlorine bleach dilution of 1:10 or a disinfectant with a product label stating that it is HIV-cidal or tuberculocidal should be used to disinfect tourniquets and items contaminated with blood or other body fluids.

23.

A. Urinary tract infections are the most prevalent of nosocomial infections.

B. Urinary tract infections are the most prevalent of nosocomial infections.

C. Urinary tract infections are the most prevalent of nosocomial infections.

D. Urinary tract infections are the most prevalent of nosocomial infections. (p. 95)

24.

A. Under the new CDC isolation guidelines, the old categories of isolation and disease-specific precautions have been collapsed into three sets of precautions that include airborne, droplet, and contact. (p. 101)

B. Under the new CDC isolation guidelines, the old categories of isolation and disease-specific precautions have been collapsed into three sets of precautions that include airborne, droplet, and contact.

C. Under the new CDC isolation guidelines, the old categories of isolation and disease-specific precautions have been collapsed into three sets of precautions that include airborne, droplet, and contact.

D. Under the new CDC isolation guidelines, the old categories of isolation and disease-specific precautions have been collapsed into three sets of precautions that include airborne, droplet, and contact.

25.

A. Standard precautions are a combination of the universal precautions and the body substance isolation. These precautions apply to blood, *all* body fluids, nonintact skin, and mucous membranes.

B. Standard precautions are a combination of the universal precautions and the body substance isolation. These precautions apply to blood, *all* body fluids, nonintact skin, and mucous membranes. (p. 102)

C. Standard precautions are a combination of the universal precautions and the body substance isolation. These precautions apply to blood, *all* body fluids, nonintact skin, and mucous membranes.

D. Standard precautions are a combination of the universal precautions and the body substance isolation. These precautions apply to blood, *all* body fluids, nonintact skin, and mucous membranes.

26.

A. Except for protective (reverse) isolation, any of the category-specific isolation precautions require that any equipment taken into the room must be left there.

B. Except for protective (reverse) isolation, any of the category-specific isolation precautions require that any equipment taken into the room must be left there.

C. Except for protective (reverse) isolation, any of the category-specific isolation precautions require that any equipment taken into the room must be left there.

D. Except for protective (reverse) isolation, any of the category-specific isolation precautions require that any equipment that is taken into the room must be left there. (p. 103)

27.

A. Tuberculosis isolation is sometimes referred to as acid-fast bacilli (AFB) isolation to protect the patient's confidentiality.

B. Tuberculosis isolation is sometimes referred to as acid-fast bacilli (AFB) isolation to protect the patient's confidentiality. (p. 105)

C. Tuberculosis isolation is sometimes referred to as acid-fast bacilli (AFB) isolation to protect the patient's confidentiality.

D. Tuberculosis isolation is sometimes referred to as acid-fast bacilli (AFB) isolation to protect the patient's confidentiality.

28.

A. Drug use is definitely a factor that affects a host's susceptibility to infection, since drug use decreases the status of the person's immune resistance. (p. 100)

B. Immunizations increase the immune response of a person to infectious diseases and decrease the chance of infections.

C. Use of disposable equipment decreases the chances of infections, since the disposable equipment is sterile or chemically clean.

D. Proper nutrition increases the host's resistance to infections.

29.

A. Tuberculosis or AFB isolation is indicated for patients with infectious tuberculosis.

B. Contact isolation was designed to prevent the spread of highly transmissible infections that do not warrant strict isolation but are conveyed primarily by direct contact such as patients infected with antibiotic-resistant microorganisms. (pp. 104–105)

C. Enteric isolation is indicated for patients with infections that are transmitted by ingestion of the pathogen *Salmonella*.

D. Enteric isolation is indicated for patients with infections that are transmitted by ingestion of the pathogen *Shigella*.

30.

A. If a worker has rubella, he/she must not work for a minimum of 5 days or until the rash clears.

B. If a worker has chicken pox, he/she must not work for 7 days after eruption first appears, provided lesions are dry and crusted when he/she returns.

C. If a worker has measles, he/she must remain off work a minimum of four days or until the rash clears.

D. Strep throat (Group A) requires that the employee be placed on appropriate antibiotics for 24 hours before he/she may come to work. (p. 98)

31.

A. Objects that can harbor infectious agents and transmit infection are called fomites. (p. 100)

B. 70% isopropyl alcohol is an antiseptic.

C. Hexachlorophene is an antiseptic.

D. Iodine for blood culture collection is an antiseptic.

32.

A. After gowning, a mask (if necessary) may be put over the nose and mouth. Then, gloves should be put on and pulled over the ends of gown sleeves.

B. After gowning, a mask (if necessary) may be put over the nose and mouth. Then, gloves should be put on and pulled over the ends of gown sleeves.

C. After gowning, a mask (if necessary) may be put over the nose and mouth. Then, gloves should be put on and pulled over the ends of gown sleeves.

D. After gowning, a mask (if necessary) may be put over the nose and mouth. Then, gloves should be put on and pulled over the ends of gown sleeves. (pp. 115–116)

33.

A. Handwashing is the most important procedure in the prevention of disease transmission in health care facilities. In any isolation procedures, it should be the first and last step.

B. Handwashing is the most important procedure in the prevention of disease transmission in health care facilities. In any isolation procedures, it should be the first and last step.

C. Handwashing is the most important procedure in the prevention of disease transmission in health care facilities. In any isolation procedures, it should be the first and last step. (p. 112)

D. Handwashing is the most important procedure in the prevention of disease transmission in health care facilities. In any isolation procedures, it should be the first and last step.

34.

A. *Campylobacter* infections require enteric isolation.

B. *Vibrio* infections require enteric isolation.

C. Respiratory isolation is required for patients with infections that may be transmitted over a short distance through the air. An example of such an infection is mumps. (p. 104)

D. *Clostridium difficile* infections require enteric isolation.

35.

A. Drainage/secretion isolation is required after surgery or if a patient is admitted with a skin infection. It is required only for a recognized source of infection.

B. Enteric isolation is required for patients with recognizable infections that are transmitted by ingestion of a pathogen.

C. Complete isolation is required for patients having a recognizable contagious disease such as rabies or chicken pox.

D. Standard precautions are designed to reduce the risk of transmission of microorganisms from both recognized and unrecognized sources of infection in health care facilities. (p. 102)

36.

A. The Joint Commission on Accreditation of Healthcare Organizations (JCAHO) requires the development and implementation of an infection control program in a health care facility. (p. 94)

B. The Joint Commission on Accreditation of Healthcare Organizations (JCAHO) requires the development and implementation of an infection control program in a health care facility.

C. The Joint Commission on Accreditation of Healthcare Organizations (JCAHO) requires the development and implementation of an infection control program in a health care facility.

D. The Joint Commission on Accreditation of Healthcare Organizations (JCAHO) requires the development and implementation of an infection control program in a health care facility.

37.

A. The classification of infections according to prevalence rates is referred to as infection control surveillance. (p. 95)

B. Nosocomial infections are those acquired after admission to a health care facility.

C. The classification of infections according to prevalence rates is referred to as infection control surveillance.

D. The classification of infections according to prevalence rates is referred to as infection control surveillance.

38.

A. The Occupational Safety and Health Administration (OSHA), an agency of the U.S. Department of Labor, requires employers to provide measures that will protect workers exposed to biological hazards.

B. The Occupational Safety and Health Administration (OSHA), an agency of the U.S. Department of Labor, requires employers to provide measures that will protect workers exposed to biological hazards.

C. The Occupational Safety and Health Administration (OSHA), an agency of the U.S. Department of Labor, requires employers to provide measures that will protect workers exposed to biological hazards. (p. 108)

D. The Occupational Safety and Health Administration (OSHA), an agency of the U.S. Department of Labor, requires employers to provide measures that will protect workers exposed to biological hazards.

39.

A. Body substance isolation (BSI) is a newer type of isolation that focuses on the isolation of potentially infectious moist body substances.

B. Body substance isolation (BSI) is a newer type of isolation that focuses on the isolation of potentially infectious moist body substances.

C. Body substance isolation (BSI) is a newer type of isolation that focuses on the isolation of potentially infectious moist body substances. (p. 105)

D. Body substance isolation (BSI) is a newer type of isolation that focuses on the isolation of potentially infectious moist body substances.

40.

A. Laboratories have a high incidence of hepatitis B, tuberculosis, tularamia, and Rocky Mountain spotted fever.

B. Laboratories have a high incidence of hepatitis B, tuberculosis, tularamia, and Rocky Mountain spotted fever. (p. 111)

C. Laboratories have a high incidence of hepatitis B, tuberculosis, tularamia, and Rocky Mountain spotted fever.

D. Laboratories have a high incidence of hepatitis B, tuberculosis, tularamia, and Rocky Mountain spotted fever.

41.

A. If an accident occurs, such as a needlestick, the health care provider should immediately cleanse the area with isopropyl alcohol and apply a bandage.

B. If an accident occurs, such as a needlestick, the health care provider should immediately cleanse the area with isopropyl alcohol and apply a bandage.

C. If an accident occurs, such as a needlestick, the health care provider should immediately cleanse the area with isopropyl alcohol and apply an adhesive bandage. (p. 108)

D. If an accident occurs, such as a needlestick, the health care provider should immediately cleanse the area with isopropyl alcohol and apply a bandage.

5 Safety and First Aid

chapter objectives

Upon completion of Chapter 5, the learner is responsible for the following:

➤ Discuss safety awareness for health care workers.

➤ Explain the measures that should be taken for fire, electrical, radiation, mechanical, and chemical safety in a health care facility.

➤ Describe the essential elements of a disaster emergency plan for a health care facility.

➤ Explain the safety policies and procedures that must be followed in all phases of specimen collection and transportation.

➤ Describe the safe use of equipment in health care facilities.

DIRECTIONS Each of the questions or incomplete statements below is followed by four suggested answers or completions. Select **one answer** that is best in each case.

 KNOWLEDGE LEVEL = 1

1. Safe working conditions must be ensured by the employer and have been mandated by law under the:
   A. Occupational Safety and Health Administration standards
   B. Institutional Safety and Health Act
   C. Health Care Facility Institutional Safety Act
   D. Health Care Facility and Occupational Safety Act

 KNOWLEDGE LEVEL = 1

2. The health care provider is most likely to encounter which of the following hazards upon entering the nuclear medicine department to obtain a blood specimen from a patient?
   A. a fire hazard
   B. a radiation hazard
   C. a mechanical hazard
   D. an electrical hazard

 KNOWLEDGE LEVEL = 1

3. If a health care provider is in an area of the health care facility where a fire starts, she or he should *first*:
   A. attempt to extinguish the fire, using the proper equipment
   B. pull the lever in the fire alarm box
   C. close all the doors and windows before leaving the area
   D. block the entrances so that others will not enter the fire area

 KNOWLEDGE LEVEL = 1

4. For safety in the health care facility, which of the following should *not* occur?
   A. Needles, syringes, and lancets should be disposed of in a special sturdy container.
   B. Liquid waste should be discarded rapidly.
   C. The specimen collection area should be disinfected periodically according to the clinical laboratory schedule.
   D. The patients' specimens should be covered at all times during transportation.

 KNOWLEDGE LEVEL = 2

5. Which of the following organizations regulates the disposal of waste?
   A. EPA
   B. NCCLS
   C. NFPA
   D. JCAHO

 KNOWLEDGE LEVEL = 1

6. The first step in controlling severe bleeding is to:
   A. send for medical assistance
   B. start cardiopulmonary resuscitation
   C. apply pressure directly over the wound or venipuncture site
   D. make the individual lie down and apply pressure to the person's forehead

KNOWLEDGE LEVEL = 2

7. If a health care provider is caught in a fire in the health care institution, she or he should *not*:
    A. run
    B. close all the doors and windows before leaving the area
    C. attempt to extinguish the fire if it is small
    D. call the assigned fire number

 KNOWLEDGE LEVEL = 1

8. If a chemical is spilled onto a health care worker, she or he should first:
    A. rub vigorously with one hand
    B. wait to see whether it starts to burn the skin
    C. rinse the area with a neutral chemical
    D. rinse the area with water

 KNOWLEDGE LEVEL = 2

9. Chemicals that are defined as "explosive flammables" must be stored:
    A. in a separate storage room
    B. in small carrying containers
    C. on a high shelf away from light and heat
    D. in an explosion-proof or fireproof room or cabinet

 KNOWLEDGE LEVEL = 2

10. According to the hazard labeling system developed by NFPA, the yellow quadrant of the diamond indicates a:
    A. flammability hazard
    B. health hazard
    C. instability hazard
    D. specific hazard

 KNOWLEDGE LEVEL = 2

11. The hazardous labeling system developed by the NFPA has the blue quadrant of the diamond to indicate a:
    A. flammability hazard
    B. health hazard
    C. instability hazard
    D. specific hazard

 KNOWLEDGE LEVEL = 2

12. If an electrical accident occurs involving electrical shock to an employee or a patient, the *first* thing that the health care worker should do is:
    A. move the victim
    B. shut off electrical power
    C. start CPR
    D. place a blanket over the victim

 KNOWLEDGE LEVEL = 1

13. What are the major principles of self-protection from radiation exposure?
    A. distance, combustibility, and shielding
    B. time, distance, and shielding
    C. anticorrosive, shielding, and distance
    D. combustibility, anticorrosive, and distance

 KNOWLEDGE LEVEL = 2

14. MSDSs must be supplied to employees according to the:
    A. Hazard Communication Standard (29 CFR 1910.1200)
    B. Environmental Protection Agency
    C. NFPA
    D. CDC

KNOWLEDGE LEVEL = 2

15. The first step in giving mouth-to-mouth resuscitation is to:

   A. open the airway by checking for obstructions

   B. listen and feel for return of air from the victim's mouth

   C. determine whether the victim is conscious by gently shaking the victim and yelling, "Are you okay?"

   D. look for the victim's chest to rise and fall

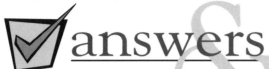
answers & rationales

1.

A. Safe working conditions must be ensured by the employer and have been mandated by law under the Occupational Safety and Health Administration (OSHA) standards. (p. 124)

B. Safe working conditions must be ensured by the employer and have been mandated by law under the Occupational Safety and Health Administration (OSHA) standards.

C. Safe working conditions must be ensured by the employer and have been mandated by law under the Occupational Safety and Health Administration (OSHA) standards.

D. Safe working conditions must be ensured by the employer and have been mandated by law under the Occupational Safety and Health Administration (OSHA) standards.

2.

A. The health care provider is most likely to encounter a radiation hazard when he or she enters the nuclear medicine department to obtain a blood specimen from a patient.

B. The health care provider is most likely to encounter a radiation hazard when he or she enters the nuclear medicine department to obtain a blood specimen from a patient. (pp. 130–131)

C. The health care provider is most likely to encounter a radiation hazard when he or she enters the nuclear medicine department to obtain a blood specimen from a patient.

D. The health care provider is most likely to encounter a radiation hazard when he or she enters the nuclear medicine department to obtain a blood specimen from a patient.

3.

A. If the fire is small, attempt to extinguish it, using the proper equipment only after first pulling the lever in the fire alarm box.

B. If a health care provider is in an area of the health care facility where a fire starts, he or she should *first* pull the lever in the fire alarm box. (p. 129)

C. If the fire is small, attempt to extinguish it, using the proper equipment only after first pulling the lever in the fire alarm box.

D. If the fire is small, attempt to extinguish it, using the proper equipment only after first pulling the lever in the fire alarm box.

4.

A. Needles, syringes, and lancets should be disposed of in a special sturdy container.

B. Liquid waste must be disposed of gently so that the liquid does not splash onto other objects or into the health care provider's eyes. (p. 126)

C. The specimen collection area should be disinfected periodically according to the clinical laboratory schedule.

D. The patients' specimens should be covered at all times during transportation.

5.

A. EPA as well as OSHA, state, and local regulations and laws regulate the disposal of waste. (p. 126)

B. The National Committee for Clinical Laboratory Standards (NCCLS) provides standards for disposal of biological and chemical wastes but does not actually regulate the waste disposal.

C. The National Fire Protection Association (NFPA) oversees fire safety, not biological waste disposal.

D. The Joint Commission on Accreditation of Healthcare Organizations provides accrediting standards for disposal of biological waste but does not regulate biological waste disposal.

6.

A. Sending for medical assistance should be the second step in controlling severe bleeding.

B. Starting cardiopulmonary resuscitation (CPR) should occur if the person's breathing movements stop or the person's lips, tongue, and fingernails become blue.

C. The first step in controlling severe bleeding is to apply pressure directly over the wound or venipuncture site. (p. 135)

D. The first step in controlling severe bleeding is to apply pressure directly over the wound or venipuncture site.

7.

A. If a health care provider is caught in a fire in the health care institution, she or he should *not* run. (p. 130)

B. If a health care provider is caught in a fire in the health care institution, she or he should close all doors and windows before leaving the area.

C. If a health care provider is caught in a fire in the health care institution, she or he should attempt to extinguish the fire if it is small.

D. If a health care provider is caught in a fire in the health care institution, she or he should call the assigned fire number.

8.

A. The victim of a chemical accident must immediately rinse the affected area with water for at least 15 minutes after removing contaminated clothing.

B. The victim of a chemical accident must immediately rinse the affected area with water for at least 15 minutes after removing contaminated clothing.

C. The victim of a chemical accident must immediately rinse the affected area with water for at least 15 minutes after removing contaminated clothing.

D. The victim of a chemical accident must immediately rinse the affected area with water for at least 15 minutes after removing contaminated clothing. (p. 133)

9.

A. Any explosive flammables must be stored in an explosion-proof or fireproof room or a cabinet.

B. Any explosive flammables must be stored in an explosion-proof or fireproof room or a cabinet.

C. Any explosive flammables must be stored in an explosion-proof or fireproof room or a cabinet.

D. Any explosive flammables must be stored in an explosion-proof or fireproof room or cabinet. (p. 133)

10.

A. The yellow quadrant of the NFPA's 0 to 4 hazard rating system indicates an instability hazard.

B. The yellow quadrant of the NFPA's 0 to 4 hazard rating system indicates an instability hazard.

C. The yellow quadrant of the NFPA's 0 to 4 hazard rating system indicates an instability hazard. (p. 132)

D. The yellow quadrant of the NFPA's 0 to 4 hazard rating system indicates an instability hazard.

11.

A. The blue quadrant of the NFPA's 0 to 4 hazard rating system indicates a health hazard.

B. The blue quadrant of the NFPA's 0 to 4 hazard rating system indicates a health hazard. (p. 132)

C. The blue quadrant of the NFPA's 0 to 4 hazard rating system indicates a health hazard.

D. The blue quadrant of the NFPA's 0 to 4 hazard rating system indicates a health hazard.

12.

A. If an electrical accident occurs involving electrical shock for an employee or a patient, the *first* thing that the health care worker should do is shut off electrical power.

B. If an electrical accident occurs involving electrical shock for an employee or a patient, the *first* thing that the health care worker should do is shut off electrical power. (p. 130)

C. Medical assistance should be called and cardiopulmonary resuscitation (CPR) started immediately *after* the electrical power is shut off.

D. A blanket should be placed over the electrocuted victim after the electrical power is shut off.

13.

A. The three cardinal principles of self-protection from radiation exposure are time, shielding, and distance.

B. The three cardinal principles of self-protection from radiation exposure are time, shielding, and distance. (p. 130)

C. The three cardinal principles of self-protection from radiation exposure are time, shielding, and distance.

D. The three cardinal principles of self-protection from radiation exposure are time, shielding, and distance.

14.

A. OSHA amended the Hazard Communication Standard (29 CFR 1910.1200) to include health care facilities. Thus labels for hazardous chemicals must (1) provide a warning (e.g. corrosive), (2) explain the nature of the hazard, (3) state special precautions to eliminate risks, and (4) explain first-aid treatment in the event of a leak, a chemical spill, or other exposure to the chemical. (p. 132)

B. OSHA amended the Hazard Communication Standard (29 CFR 1910.1200) to include health care facilities. Thus labels for hazardous chemicals must (1) provide a warning (e.g. corrosive), (2) explain the nature of the hazard, (3) state special precautions to eliminate risks, and (4) explain first-aid treatment in the event of a leak, a chemical spill, or other exposure to the chemical.

C. OSHA amended the Hazard Communication Standard (29 CFR 1910.1200) to include health care facilities. Thus labels for hazardous chemicals must (1) provide a warning (e.g. corrosive), (2) explain the nature of the hazard, (3) state special precautions to eliminate risks, and (4) explain first-aid treatment in the event of a leak, a chemical spill, or other exposure to the chemical.

D. OSHA amended the Hazard Communication Standard (29 CFR 1910.1200) to include health care facilities. Thus labels for hazardous chemicals must (1) provide a warning (e.g. corrosive), (2) explain the nature of the hazard, (3) state special precautions to eliminate risks, and (4) explain first-aid treatment in the event of a leak, a chemical spill, or other exposure to the chemical.

15.

A. Opening the airway by checking for obstructions is the third step in giving mouth-to-mouth resuscitation. The first step in giving mouth-to-mouth resuscitation is to determine whether the victim is conscious by gently shaking the victim and yelling, "Are you okay?"

B. The first step in giving mouth-to-mouth resuscitation is to determine whether the victim is conscious by gently shaking the victim and yelling, "Are you okay?"

C. The first step in giving mouth-to-mouth resuscitation is to determine whether the victim is conscious by gently shaking the victim and yelling, "Are you okay?" (p. 135)

D. The first step in giving mouth-to-mouth resuscitation is to determine whether the victim is conscious by gently shaking the victim and yelling, "Are you okay?"

6 Specimen Documentation and Transportation

chapter objectives

Upon completion of Chapter 6, the learner is responsible for the following:

➤ Describe the basic components of a clinical or medical record.

➤ Identify six ways to enhance the intralaboratory communication network.

➤ Describe essential elements of requisition and report forms.

➤ Name three methods that are commonly used to transport specimens.

➤ Name areas or departments that usually receive laboratory reports.

DIRECTIONS Each of the questions or incomplete statements below is followed by suggested answers or completions. Select **one answer** that is best in each case.

 KNOWLEDGE LEVEL = 1

1. A patient's medical record can best be described as:
   A. a legal document that provides a chronological log of care
   B. a legal document that is available only to the patient's physician
   C. the procedure for a selected care plan
   D. public information that may be disclosed during a financial inquiry

 KNOWLEDGE LEVEL = 1

2. JCAHO is:
   A. a proficiency testing agency
   B. an accrediting agency for health care facilities
   C. an agency that administers certifications
   D. a governmental agency that administers Medicare

 KNOWLEDGE LEVEL = 1

3. The Hazard Communication Standard relates to:
   A. procedures and documentation regarding hazardous substances
   B. quality-control procedures
   C. attendance and behavior policies
   D. instrument and maintenance records for equipment

 KNOWLEDGE LEVEL = 1

4. Bar codes can be used in health care for patient identification purposes. Which of the following characterizes how bar codes are interpreted?
   A. The bars indicate pricing for laboratory procedures.
   B. Light and dark bands of varying widths represent alphanumeric symbols.
   C. They contain the name of the institution.
   D. They reveal the nature of each specimen.

 KNOWLEDGE LEVEL = 1

5. The most efficient and accurate way of making labels for specimens is by:
   A. imprinting the physician's orders directly from the Kardex
   B. printing from a computerized system
   C. manually labeling the specimens as each one is drawn
   D. none of the above

 KNOWLEDGE LEVEL = 1

6. Serum should be transported to the laboratory for testing and separated from blood cells within which of the following time periods to prevent erroneous test results?
   A. 5 hours
   B. 4 hours
   C. 2 hours
   D. 5 minutes

KNOWLEDGE LEVEL = 2

7. Why should one use an airtight container with icy water to transport an arterial specimen for blood gas analysis?
   A. It decreases the loss of gases from the specimen.
   B. It promotes coagulation.
   C. It aids in the instrumentation phase of the testing process.
   D. It increases the oxygen content in the specimen.

 KNOWLEDGE LEVEL = 1

8. PROs use documentation in the medical records for which of the following purposes?
   A. to check the quality of care and medical stability of patients
   B. to check for unnecessary procedures and tests
   C. to evaluate whether the patient's charges are warranted
   D. all of the above

 KNOWLEDGE LEVEL = 1

9. Characteristics of the documentation in a medical record include which of the following?
   A. accurate
   B. complete
   C. objective and factual
   D. all of the above

 KNOWLEDGE LEVEL = 1

10. The basic format for most technical procedures includes:
    A. name and title of the procedure
    B. description of the method and its clinical significance

   C. specimen requirements, reference ranges, and quality-control steps
   D. all of the above

 KNOWLEDGE LEVEL = 1

11. Confidential patient information includes:
    A. clinical laboratory results
    B. the name of the phlebotomist who draws a specimen
    C. the name of the laboratory supervisor
    D. none of the above

 KNOWLEDGE LEVEL = 2

12. Assays that require a chilled specimen include:
    A. gastrin, ammonia, and lactic acid
    B. renin, catecholamine, and parathyroid hormone determinations
    C. blood gases and PT, PTT
    D. all of the above

 KNOWLEDGE LEVEL = 2

13. To chill a blood specimen as it is transported, the health care worker should use:
    A. tepid water
    B. a small freezer unit
    C. icy water
    D. frozen blocks of ice

 KNOWLEDGE LEVEL = 2

14. Specimens that require protection from light include those for:
    A. CBC, diff, and platelet counts
    B. PT and PTTs
    C. bilirubin and porphyrin
    D. none of the above

KNOWLEDGE LEVEL = 2

15. Specimens that require warming to body temperature are those for:
    A. CBC, diff, and platelet counts
    B. PT and PTTs
    C. bilirubin and porphyrin
    D. cold agglutinins and cryofibrinogen

 KNOWLEDGE LEVEL = 1

16. Laboratory reports containing test results should go through which of the following protocols?
    A. Release results immediately upon completion of the testing process.
    B. Confirm results, date the release of results, and send a permanent copy to the clinical record.
    C. Call the results to a physician.
    D. Fax the results immediately to the patient.

 KNOWLEDGE LEVEL = 1

17. Specimens other than blood may need to be transported by health care workers using special handling procedures. In the laboratory department, these specimens may include:
    A. human or animal feces
    B. body fluids
    C. tissues
    D. all of the above

 KNOWLEDGE LEVEL = 1

18. In designing a report form for laboratory results, what key elements must be included?
    A. patient and physician identification
    B. date and time of collection
    C. reference ranges
    D. all of the above

 KNOWLEDGE LEVEL = 1

19. The use of log sheets in a specimen collection area serves to:
    A. provide a record of specimens collected
    B. keep confidential information available
    C. keep track of employee productivity
    D. track quality control of supplies/reagents

 KNOWLEDGE LEVEL = 1

20. Which of the following factors should be considered when pneumatic tube systems are used for transporting specimens?
    A. mechanical reliability and distance of transport
    B. speed of carrier and landing mechanism
    C. effect on the chemical and cellular components of specimens
    D. all of the above

 KNOWLEDGE LEVEL = 1

21. The most reliable labeling method for avoiding transcription errors in specimen collection is:
    A. handwritten labels with careful attention to detail
    B. computerized labels using bar codes
    C. addressograph machine
    D. none of the above

 KNOWLEDGE LEVEL = 1

22. Bar codes represent:
    A. light and dark bands of varying widths
    B. alphanumeric symbols
    C. specific codes for numbers and letters
    D. all of the above

KNOWLEDGE LEVEL = 1

23. Quality control records include information about:
    A. hazards associated with the use of a reagent or supplies
    B. proper use and storage information
    C. expiration dates and stability information
    D. all of the above

 KNOWLEDGE LEVEL = 1

24. Continuing education for phlebotomists may include:
    A. fire safety
    B. standard precautions
    C. radiation safety
    D. all of the above

 KNOWLEDGE LEVEL = 1

25. When a phlebotomist has failed to draw a blood specimen after two attempts, what should be done?
    A. Call the doctor.
    B. Call the nurse immediately.
    C. Try one more time.
    D. none of the above

 KNOWLEDGE LEVEL = 1

26. If a hospital patient is unavailable at the time a phlebotomist arrives to collect a blood specimen, what should be done?
    A. Continue with other blood collections until complete, then check back.
    B. Leave the supplies on the patient's hospital bed for someone else.
    C. Track down the patient.
    D. none of the above

 KNOWLEDGE LEVEL = 1

27. If a patient refuses to have a simple venipuncture, what should be done?
    A. Continue with other blood collections until complete, then check back.
    B. Leave the supplies on the patient's hospital bed for someone else to try.
    C. Leave the patient and notify a nurse.
    D. Try to convince a patient that it must be done.

 KNOWLEDGE LEVEL = 1

28. Bar codes can be used for:
    A. patient names
    B. patient identification numbers
    C. laboratory test numbers
    D. all of the above

 KNOWLEDGE LEVEL = 1

29. Preanalytical errors are errors that happen before the actual laboratory testing phase. Transportation variables that may cause such errors include:
    A. tube breakage
    B. inadequate centrifugation
    C. inadequate volume in the test tube
    D. patient stress and anxiety

 KNOWLEDGE LEVEL = 1

30. Preanalytical errors are errors that happen before the actual laboratory testing phase. Patient variables that may cause such errors include:
    A. tube breakage
    B. inadequate centrifugation
    C. inadequate volume in the test tube
    D. patient stress and anxiety

KNOWLEDGE LEVEL = 2

31. Preanalytical errors are those that happen before the actual laboratory testing phase. Specimen processing variables that may cause errors include:
    A. excessive shaking or mixing
    B. inadequate centrifugation
    C. exposure to heat or light
    D. all of the above

 KNOWLEDGE LEVEL = 1

32. An infection control manual normally contains which of the following policies/procedures?
    A. isolation methods
    B. decontamination procedures
    C. hand-washing procedures
    D. all of the above

 KNOWLEDGE LEVEL = 2

Questions 33–35 relate to the following case scenario:

Mary was a medical assistant in a family health clinic with a small laboratory. She had responsibilities in several areas, including answering the phone in the laboratory, drawing blood specimens, clerical duties, and assisting with laboratory testing. One morning when the clinic was particularly busy, she was drawing blood for numerous patients and trying to process them so that they could be tested in a timely manner. When the phone rang, she was reluctant to answer it because she had almost finished processing a batch of samples. It rang several times; then she hurried to pick it up and asked the individual to "hold please." She went back to finish processing the samples and forgot the person on hold. Later she found out that the individual on hold was a doctor who was trying to request another test on a previously drawn sample.

33. What should Mary have said when she first answered the phone?
    A. "Hold for just a moment please."
    B. "Please hold while I process a few specimens so that they will not be delayed."
    C. "Hello, this is the clinic laboratory. May I help you?"
    D. "Hello, I am sorry that I cannot assist you now. Please call back."

 KNOWLEDGE LEVEL = 2

34. From what type of additional training would Mary benefit?
    A. effective customer service
    B. how to place a caller on hold
    C. effective communication
    D. all of the above

 KNOWLEDGE LEVEL = 2

35. To improve communication and enhance the flow of information, what other types of technology should be considered to assist the laboratory in the processing of specimens?
    A. a fax machine for receiving requests
    B. bar coding specimens for rapid and efficient processing
    C. a speakerphone
    D. all of the above

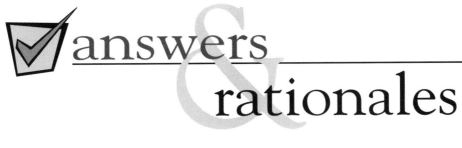

answers & rationales

1.

A. The medical or clinical record is the definitive legal document that provides a chronological log of the patient's care. (pp. 144–145)

B. The medical record is a legal document that is available not only to the patient's physician, but also to other members of the patient's health care team. Documentation in the medical record provides proof of the quality of care given.

C. The medical record may include a procedure for a selected care plan but also includes many other components related to the care of the patient.

D. The medical record is a confidential, private record and is not subject to review by the general public. Information may not be disclosed during a financial inquiry unless the hospital or patient gives permission.

2.

A. Proficiency testing refers to testing laboratory samples provided by an independent agency to assess the accuracy of test results compared to other clinical laboratories. Laboratories subscribe to proficiency testing programs to comply with CLIA and to assess their accuracy and precision. JCAHO does not provide laboratory samples for proficiency testing.

B. JCAHO is an accrediting agency for health care organizations. Among other requirements, they have specific standards for documentation in each patient's medical record. They usually include an assessment, a plan of care, medical orders, progress notes, and a discharge summary. (p. 144)

C. JCAHO does not administer certification examinations.

D. JCAHO does not administer Medicare and is not affiliated with the government.

3.

A. The Hazard Communication Standard refers to guidelines designed to protect workers from hazardous substances. (p. 150)

B. Quality-control procedures relate to the conduct of diagnostic laboratory testing. They usually include information about hazards, proper use, storage and handling of reagents used in laboratory testing, stability of the chemical, expiration dates, and indications for measuring the precision and accuracy of analytic processes.

C. Attendance and behavior policies are usually listed in administrative procedure manuals and are usually covered during the orientation period for new employees.

D. The history and performance records of clinical laboratory instruments are kept in instrument and maintenance manuals for the clinical laboratory.

4.

A. Bar codes are most commonly used for patient identification during the specimen collection process; however, they might also be used for billing codes, laboratory test codes, inventory records, and sample aliquots.

B. Bar codes represent a series of light and dark bands of varying widths that represent alphanumeric symbols. (p. 154)

C. Refer to A.

D. Refer to A.

5.

A. Imprinting the physician's orders directly from the Kardex is not the most accurate or efficient method of labeling specimens.

B. The most accurate method to generate specimen labels is by using computerized systems. Computerization of the collection process can significantly decrease errors because data are continually being checked against the computer files, and authorized individuals can add to and receive designated information. (p. 159)

C. Manually labeling the specimens as each one is drawn is not as accurate or efficient as using computer-generated labels because it is prone to transcription errors.

D. "None of the above" is not the correct answer.

6.

A. Five hours would result in excessive delays after blood collection, resulting in glycolytic action from the blood cells interfering with the analysis of several constituents, including glucose, calcitonin, aldosterone, phosphorus, and enzymes.

B. Four hours would result in excessive delays after blood collection, resulting in glycolytic action from the blood cells interfering with the analysis of several constituents, including glucose, aldosterone, phosphorus, and enzymes.

C. Blood specimens should always be transported to the clinical laboratory for testing as soon as possible, ideally within 45 minutes but no more than 2 hours from the time of collection so that the serum or plasma can be separated from the blood cells. Once separated, serum may remain at room temperature, be refrigerated, be stored in a dark place, or be frozen, depending on the test methodology. Serum should be covered to prevent evaporation, which can cause some constituents to become more concentrated and thus cause erroneous results. (p. 160)

D. Five minutes is not enough time to allow the blood to clot adequately and is usually not a realistic transport time for most clinical specimens with the exception of a laboratory located at the site of collection or a point-of-service scenario.

7.

A. An airtight container and icy water decrease the loss of gases from the specimen. (p. 160)

B. Coagulation is not promoted by icy water or the airtight container, nor is it desired for a blood gas analysis.

C. The container and icy water help to ensure an accurate and reliable result due to a properly handled specimen but do not have an effect on the instrumentation phase of testing.

D. The container and icy water do not increase the oxygen content in the specimen.

8.

A. Physician review organizations (PROs) use documentation in the clinical record to evaluate the quality of care for specific indicators such as nosocomial infections, medical stability of the patient, unnecessary procedures and tests, adequate discharge planning, and the occurrence of avoidable discomfort or death. PROs can impose fines or sanctions or deny reimbursements if care delivered seems inappropriate.

B. Physician review organizations (PROs) use documentation in the clinical record to evaluate the quality of care for specific indicators such as nosocomial infections, medical stability of the patient, unnecessary procedures and tests, adequate discharge planning, and the occurrence of avoidable discomfort or death. PROs can impose fines or sanctions or deny reimbursements if care delivered seems inappropriate.

C. Physician review organizations (PROs) use documentation in the clinical record to evaluate the quality of care for specific indicators such as nosocomial infections, medical stability of the patient, unnecessary procedures and tests, adequate discharge planning, and the occurrence of avoidable discomfort or death. PROs can impose fines or sanctions or deny reimbursements if care delivered seems inappropriate.

D. Physician review organizations (PROs) use documentation in the clinical record to evaluate the quality of care for specific indicators such as nosocomial infections, medical stability of the patient, unnecessary procedures and tests, adequate discharge planning, and the occurrence of avoidable discomfort or death. PROs can impose fines or sanctions or deny reimbursements if care delivered seems inappropriate. (p. 144)

9.

A. Documentation in the clinical record should be accurate, complete, objective, and factual. Accuracy refers to recording the precise facts, not opinions or assumptions, and should never be changed or falsified. Complete notes include the exact time of the procedure and identify other relevant sources of information about the process. Objectivity refers to being factual about the situation or process. It means not assigning blame or including extraneous facts that are unrelated to the patient's care.

B. Documentation in the clinical record should be accurate, complete, objective, and factual. Accuracy refers to recording the precise facts, not opinions or assumptions, and should never be changed or falsified. Complete notes include the exact time of the procedure and identify other relevant sources of information about the process. Objectivity refers to being factual about the situation or process. It means not assigning blame or including extraneous facts that are unrelated to the patient's care.

C. Documentation in the clinical record should be accurate, complete, objective, and factual. Accuracy refers to recording the precise facts, not opinions or assumptions, and should never be changed or falsified. Complete notes include the exact time of the procedure and identify other relevant sources of information about the process. Objectivity refers to being factual about the situation or process. It means not assigning blame or including extraneous facts that are unrelated to the patient's care.

D. Documentation in the clinical record should be accurate, complete, objective, and factual. Accuracy refers to recording the precise facts, not opinions or assumptions, and should never be changed or falsified. Complete notes include the exact time of the procedure and identify other relevant sources of information about the process. Objectivity refers to being factual about the situation or process. It means not assigning blame or including extraneous facts that are unrelated to the patient's care. (p. 145)

10.

A. The College of American Pathologists requires that technical procedures are available on-site to technical personnel who perform specimen collection procedures and laboratory assays. The format for technical procedures includes the name and title of the procedure, a description of the method, specimen requirements, procedural steps, reagents and preparation required, reference ranges, the clinical significance of the results, quality-control instructions, calculations if needed, reporting requirements, approval signatures, dates, and references.

B. The College of American Pathologists requires that technical procedures are available on-site to technical personnel who perform specimen collection procedures and laboratory assays. The format for technical procedures includes the name and title of the procedure, a description of the method, specimen requirements, procedural steps, reagents and preparation required, reference ranges, the clinical significance of the results, quality-control instructions, calculations if needed, reporting requirements, approval signatures, dates, and references.

C. The College of American Pathologists requires that technical procedures are available on-site to technical personnel who perform specimen collection procedures and laboratory assays. The format for technical procedures includes the name and title of the procedure, a description of the method, specimen requirements, procedural steps, reagents and preparation required, reference ranges, the clinical significance of the results, quality-control instructions, calculations if needed, reporting requirements, approval signatures, dates, and references.

D. The College of American Pathologists requires that technical procedures are available on-site to technical personnel who perform specimen collection procedures and laboratory assays. The format for technical procedures includes the name and title of the procedure, a description of the method, specimen requirements, procedural steps, reagents and preparation required, reference ranges, the clinical significance of the results, quality-control instructions, calculations if needed, reporting requirements, approval signatures, dates, and references. (pp. 147–149)

11.

A. All clinical documents, including laboratory results, are considered confidential. In addition, communications between the patient and a physician are considered privileged in most states and are also to be treated as confidential information. Violations of a patient's confidentiality can result in legal action. (p. 152)

B. The name of the phlebotomist who draws a blood specimen is not considered confidential information. In fact, the patient has a right to know the name of the individual performing the procedure.

C. The name of the laboratory supervisor is not considered confidential information.

D. "None of the above" is an incorrect answer.

12.

A. Specimens that may require chilling include those being tested for gastrin, ammonia, lactic acid, renin, catecholamine, parathyroid hormone, prothrombin time (PT), partial thromboplastin time (PTT), glucagon, and blood gas analyses.

B. Specimens that may require chilling include those being tested for gastrin, ammonia, lactic acid, renin, catecholamine, parathyroid hormone, prothrombin time (PT), partial thromboplastin time (PTT), glucagon, and blood gas analyses.

C. Specimens that may require chilling include those being tested for gastrin, ammonia, lactic acid, renin, catecholamine, parathyroid hormone, prothrombin time (PT), partial thromboplastin time (PTT), glucagon, and blood gas analyses.

D. Specimens that may require chilling include those being tested for gastrin, ammonia, lactic acid, renin, catecholamine, parathyroid hormone, prothrombin time (PT), partial thromboplastin time (PTT), glucagon, and blood gas analyses. (p. 160)

13.

A. Tepid water is lukewarm and will not keep the specimen cool.

B. A freezer unit may actually freeze the specimen causing loss of its integrity and erroneous results.

C. Icy water or slushy water will keep the specimen cool and will not freeze it. (p. 160)

D. Frozen blocks of ice may also freeze the specimen during transport.

14.

A. Specimens for CBC, diff, and platelet counts are not light sensitive and do not need to be protected in a special manner.

B. Specimens for PT and PTTs are not light sensitive and do not need to be protected in a special manner.

C. Bilirubin and porphyrin are light sensitive and decompose if exposed to light. Specimens (blood or urine) being tested for these constituents should be protected from bright light with aluminum foil wrapping. (p. 160)

D. "None of the above" is not a correct answer.

15.

A. Specimens being tested for CBC, diff, and platelet counts do not require warming.

B. Specimens being tested for PT and PTTs do not require warming.

C. Specimens being tested for bilirubin and porphyrin do not require warming.

D. Specimens that require warming to body temperature, 37°C, include those for testing cold agglutinins and cryofibrinogen. These special cases require a heat block for transportation and handling purposes. (p. 161)

16.

A. Results should not be released immediately upon completion of the testing process.

B. The JCAHO and CAP state that laboratory results should be confirmed, dated, and a copy sent to the clinical record. (p. 164)

C. Calling the results to a physician is important if it was a "stat" request.

D. Faxing the results immediately to the patient is never appropriate without prior approval and documentation.

17.

A. Specimens such as human or animal feces; blood; body fluids such as spinal fluid, pleural fluid, or sputum; or biopsy tissues may need to be transported to reference or research laboratories. In packing or receiving one of these specimens, a special transport container must be used, with special attention to preventing leakage, temperature and pressure changes during transport, mislabeling, and breakage.

B. Specimens such as human or animal feces; blood; body fluids such as spinal fluid, pleural fluid, or sputum; or biopsy tissues may need to be transported to reference or research laboratories. In packing or receiving one of these specimens, a special transport container must be used, with special attention to preventing leakage, temperature and pressure changes during transport, mislabeling, and breakage.

C. Specimens such as human or animal feces; blood; body fluids such as spinal fluid, pleural fluid, or sputum; or biopsy tissues may need to be transported to reference or research laboratories. In packing or receiving one of these specimens, a special transport container must be used, with special attention to preventing leakage, temperature and pressure changes during transport, mislabeling, and breakage.

D. Specimens such as human or animal feces; blood; body fluids such as spinal fluid, pleural fluid, or sputum; or biopsy tissues may need to be transported to reference or research laboratories. In packing or receiving one of these specimens, a special transport container must be used, with special attention to preventing leakage, temperature and pressure changes during transport, mislabeling, and breakage. (p. 164)

18.

A. CAP recommends that in designing a laboratory report form, the following issues should be considered: identification of patient and physician, patient location, date and time of specimen collection, source and description of specimen, precautions, packaging requirements for the specimen, understandability of the report, ability to be located in the patient's clinical record, reference ranges, and abnormal values.

B. CAP recommends that in designing a laboratory report form, the following issues should be considered: identification of patient and physician, patient location, date and time of specimen collection, source and description of specimen, precautions, packaging requirements for the specimen, understandability of the report, ability to be located in the patient's clinical record, reference ranges, and abnormal values.

C. CAP recommends that in designing a laboratory report form, the following issues should be considered: identification of patient and physician, patient location, date and time of specimen collection, source and description of specimen, precautions, packaging requirements for the specimen, understandability of the report, ability to be located in the patient's clinical record, reference ranges, and abnormal values.

D. CAP recommends that in designing a laboratory report form, the following issues should be considered: identification of patient and physician, patient location, date and time of specimen collection, source and description of specimen, precautions, packaging requirements for the specimen, understandability of the report, ability to be located in the patient's clinical record, reference ranges, and abnormal values. (p. 164)

19.

A. A log book or log sheet can serve to provide a record of specimens that have been collected throughout the day. For hospital use, a copy could be located on a nursing unit as well as in the laboratory. (p. 159)

B. The log book/sheet would not serve to keep information confidential.

C. The log book/sheet would not serve to keep track of employee productivity.

D. The log book/sheet would not serve to track quality control of supplies/reagents.

20.

A. Pneumatic tube systems can be used to transport patient records, messages, letters, bills, medications, X-rays, and laboratory specimens. In considering the system for specimen transport, the following factors are important to maintain specimen integrity: mechanical reliability, distance of transport, speed of carrier, landing mechanism, effect on the chemical and cellular components of specimens, sizes of the carriers, shock absorbency, and radius of the loops and bends in the system.

B. Pneumatic tube systems can be used to transport patient records, messages, letters, bills, medications, X-rays, and laboratory specimens. In considering the system for specimen transport, the following factors are important to maintain specimen integrity: mechanical reliability, distance of transport, speed of carrier, landing mechanism, effect on the chemical and cellular components of specimens, sizes of the carriers, shock absorbency, and radius of the loops and bends in the system.

C. Pneumatic tube systems can be used to transport patient records, messages, letters, bills, medications, X-rays, and laboratory specimens. In considering the system for specimen transport, the following factors are important to maintain specimen integrity: mechanical reliability, distance of transport, speed of carrier, landing mechanism, effect on the chemical and cellular components of specimens, sizes of the carriers, shock absorbency, and radius of the loops and bends in the system.

D. Pneumatic tube systems can be used to transport patient records, messages, letters, bills, medications, X-rays, and laboratory specimens. In considering the system for specimen transport, the following factors are important to maintain specimen integrity: mechanical reliability, distance of transport, speed of carrier, landing mechanism, effect on the chemical and cellular components of specimens, sizes of the carriers, shock absorbency, and radius of the loops and bends in the system. (p. 163)

21.

A. Handwritten labels are more prone to transcription errors.

B. Computerized labels using bar codes provide the most accurate and efficient labels that can be generated. (p. 159)

C. An addressograph machine can also be used to make labels and is generally very reliable; however, it is not as efficient or reliable as computerized bar-coded labels.

D. "None of the above" is an incorrect answer.

22.

A. Bar codes represent a series of light and dark bands of varying widths that represent specific alphanumeric symbols (numbers and letters).

B. Bar codes represent a series of light and dark bands of varying widths that represent specific alphanumeric symbols (numbers and letters).

C. Bar codes represent a series of light and dark bands of varying widths that represent specific alphanumeric symbols (numbers and letters).

D. Bar codes represent a series of light and dark bands of varying widths that represent specific alphanumeric symbols (numbers and letters). (p. 154)

23.

A. Quality-control information usually contains facts about the following: hazards associated with the use of a reagent or supplies, proper use and storage information, expiration dates and stability information, and indications for measuring the precision and accuracy of the analytical process to be involved.

B. Quality-control information usually contains facts about the following: hazards associated with the use of a reagent or supplies, proper use and storage information, expiration dates and stability information, and indications for measuring the precision and accuracy of the analytical process to be involved.

C. Quality-control information usually contains facts about the following: hazards associated with the use of a reagent or supplies, proper use and storage information, expiration dates and stability information, and indications for measuring the precision and accuracy of the analytical process to be involved.

D. Quality-control information usually contains facts about the following: hazards associated with the use of a reagent or supplies, proper use and storage information, expiration dates and stability information, and indications for measuring the precision and accuracy of the analytical process to be involved. (p. 150)

24.

A. Continuing education for phlebotomists may include universal standard precautions, fire safety, radiation safety, and many other organization-specific programs.

B. Continuing education for phlebotomists may include universal standard precautions, fire safety, radiation safety, and many other organization-specific programs.

C. Continuing education for phlebotomists may include universal standard precautions, fire safety, radiation safety, and many other organization-specific programs.

D. Continuing education for phlebotomists may include universal standard precautions, fire safety, radiation safety, and many other organization-specific programs. (p. 150)

25.

A. Calling the doctor may be necessary after consulting with other supervisory personnel.

B. Calling the nurse *immediately* may be overreacting; however, a supervisor should be notified of the situation. Procedures may vary according to each facility.

C. Each phlebotomist should be allowed only two venipuncture attempts on any patient.

D. If a phlebotomist is unable to obtain a specimen after two attempts, she or he should request help from a supervisor or nurse. The phlebotomist should not make another attempt. Most laboratories allow only one more person to try, again with no more than two attempts. (p. 148)

26.

A. If a phlebotomist is unable to collect blood when requested because a patient is unavailable, she or he should hold the request until other patients on the unit have been completed, then check back to see whether the patient is available. If not, then information should be documented about the reason the patient is unavailable, and a nurse should be notified of the situation. (p. 148)

B. Supplies should never be left on the patient's hospital bed.

C. Tracking down the patient may be appropriate in some instances; however, it may cause a loss of timing and productivity in collecting the remaining patient samples on that unit.

D. "None of the above" is an incorrect answer.

27.

A. It may not be beneficial to check back with the patient once they have refused. It is more important to notify a nurse and/or supervisor.

B. Supplies should never be left on the patient's hospital bed.

C. All patients have a right to refuse any procedure. Phlebotomists should respect this right. If a patient refuses, the best practice is to leave the patient and notify the nurse. Often, the nurse can convince the patient to cooperate; if not, document the incident and remain professional and respectful to the patient. (p. 148)

D. A phlebotomist should respect each patient's right to refuse a procedure and not try to convince a patient that it must be done.

28.

A. Bar codes have many applications in specimen identification, processing, and testing, including patient names, identification numbers, test codes, accession numbers, billing codes, and inventory records.

B. Bar codes have many applications in specimen identification, processing, and testing, including patient names, identification numbers, test codes, accession numbers, billing codes, and inventory records.

C. Bar codes have many applications in specimen identification, processing, and testing, including patient names, identification numbers, test codes, accession numbers, billing codes, and inventory records.

D. Bar codes have many applications in specimen identification, processing, and testing, including patient names, identification numbers, test codes, accession numbers, billing codes, and inventory records. (pp. 156–157)

29.

A. Transportation variables that affect the preanalytical phases of specimen handling include specimen leakage, tube breakage, and excessive shaking in the transport vehicle. (p. 146)

B. Inadequate centrifugation is considered a processing error.

C. Inadequate volume in the test tube is considered a preventable specimen variable or error that may be controlled by the phlebotomist.

D. Patient stress and anxiety are also preanalytical variables that may affect the process but are not related to the transportation of the specimen.

30.

A. Tube breakage is usually due to transportation or processing error.

B. Inadequate centrifugation is considered a processing error.

C. Inadequate volume in the test tube is controlled by the phlebotomist.

D. Patient variables that affect the preanalytical process are stress and anxiety, diurnal variations, refusal to cooperate, fasting condition, and availability. (p. 146)

31.

A. Processing variables that affect the preanalytical process include inadequate centrifugation, delays in processing, contamination of the specimen, exposure to heat or light, and excessive shaking or mixing.

B. Processing variables that affect the preanalytical process include inadequate centrifugation, delays in processing, contamination of the specimen, exposure to heat or light, and excessive shaking or mixing.

C. Processing variables that affect the preanalytical process include inadequate centrifugation, delays in processing, contamination of the specimen, exposure to heat or light, and excessive shaking or mixing.

D. Processing variables that affect the preanalytical process include inadequate centrifugation, delays in processing, contamination of the specimen, exposure to heat or light, and excessive shaking or mixing. (p. 146)

32.

A. An infection control manual normally contains procedures for handling specimens, isolation procedures, hand-washing procedures, disposal policies, and precaution signage.

B. An infection control manual normally contains procedures for handling specimens, isolation procedures, hand-washing procedures, disposal policies, and precaution signage.

C. An infection control manual normally contains procedures for handling specimens, isolation procedures, hand-washing procedures, disposal policies, and precaution signage.

D. An infection control manual normally contains procedures for handling specimens, isolation procedures, hand-washing procedures, disposal policies, and precaution signage. (p. 150)

33.

A. The caller should be greeted and acknowledged and asked whether he or she may be placed on hold. If the caller has an emergency, this gives him or her an opportunity to state it. If the caller is immediately placed on hold, the urgency or nature of the call remains unknown.

B. Refer to A.

C. Mary should have stopped her work temporarily to answer the phone or asked for assistance. If she had no assistance, she should have greeted the caller in a polite and professional manner, stated the department name, and asked how she could help. She should have restated the request or asked for clarification and documented it. (pp. 151–152)

D. This statement did not allow the caller to speak and is not appropriate.

34.

A. The telephone is the most frequently used method of live communication in any setting. It is vitally important that health care workers be aware of the procedures for operating it and the etiquette for professional dialogue. Training can include effective customer service manners, transferring calls, placing someone on hold, using an intercom system, using voice mail, organizing conference calls, using speakerphones, documenting complete messages, and appropriate greetings.

B. The telephone is the most frequently used method of live communication in any setting. It is vitally important that health care workers be aware of the procedures for operating it and the etiquette for professional dialogue. Training can include effective customer service manners, transferring calls, placing someone on hold, using an intercom system, using voice mail, organizing conference calls, using speakerphones, documenting complete messages, and appropriate greetings.

C. The telephone is the most frequently used method of live communication in any setting. It is vitally important that health care workers be aware of the procedures for operating it and the etiquette for professional dialogue. Training can include effective customer service manners, transferring calls, placing someone on hold, using an intercom system, using voice mail, organizing conference calls, using speakerphones, documenting complete messages, and appropriate greetings.

D. The telephone is the most frequently used method of live communication in any setting. It is vitally important that health care workers be aware of the procedures for operating it and the etiquette for professional dialogue. Training can include effective customer service manners, transferring calls, placing someone on hold, using an intercom system, using voice mail, organizing conference calls, using speakerphones, documenting complete messages, and appropriate greetings. (pp. 151–152)

35.

A. Many types of technology are available to enhance effective communication. Each facility needs to evaluate the cost and reliability of various products; among the communication devices that are commonly used in the specimen processing and collection areas are fax machines, speakerphones, voice mail, intercom systems, telephone headsets, bar code printers and scanners, and various types of computers.

B. Many types of technology are available to enhance effective communication. Each facility needs to evaluate the cost and reliability of various products; among the communication devices that are commonly used in the specimen processing and collection areas are fax machines, speakerphones, voice mail, intercom systems, telephone headsets, bar code printers and scanners, and various types of computers.

C. Many types of technology are available to enhance effective communication. Each facility needs to evaluate the cost and reliability of various products; among the communication devices that are commonly used in the specimen processing and collection areas are fax machines, speakerphones, voice mail, intercom systems, telephone headsets, bar code printers and scanners, and various types of computers.

D. Many types of technology are available to enhance effective communication. Each facility needs to evaluate the cost and reliability of various products; however, among the communication devices that are commonly used in the specimen processing and collection areas are fax machines, speakerphones, voice mail, intercom systems, telephone headsets, bar code printers and scanners, and various types of computers. (pp. 165–166)

SECTION III

Equipment and Procedures

7 Blood Collection Equipment

chapter objectives

Upon completion of Chapter 7, the learner is responsible for the following:

➤ List the various types of anticoagulants used in blood collection, their mechanisms for preventing blood from clotting, and the vacuum collection tube color codes for these anticoagulants.

➤ Describe the latest phlebotomy safety supplies and equipment, and evaluate their effectiveness in blood collection.

➤ Identify the various supplies that should be carried on a specimen collection tray when a skin puncture specimen must be collected.

➤ Identify the types of equipment needed to collect blood by venipuncture.

➤ Describe the special precautions that should be taken and the techniques that should be used when various types of specimens must be transported to the clinical laboratory.

DIRECTIONS Each of the questions or incomplete statements below is followed by four suggested answers or completions. Select **one answer** that is best in each case.

 KNOWLEDGE LEVEL = 1

1. Which of the following is a capillary blood collection system?
    A. Microtome
    B. S-Monovette
    C. Safety-Gard Phlebotomy System
    D. Samplette blood collector

 KNOWLEDGE LEVEL = 1

2. Chromosome analysis requires whole blood collected in a:
    A. green-topped tube
    B. red-topped tube
    C. gray-topped tube
    D. light blue-topped tube

 KNOWLEDGE LEVEL = 2

3. The vials shown in Figure 7.1 are used in the collection of:
    A. microscopy specimens
    B. clinical chemistry specimens
    C. clinical immunology specimens
    D. microbiology specimens

 KNOWLEDGE LEVEL = 1

4. Lithium heparin is a suitable anticoagulant for which of the following studies?
    A. erythrocyte sedimentation rate
    B. zinc level
    C. glucose level
    D. lithium level

FIGURE 7.1.

(Courtesy of Becton-Dickinson Diagnostic Instrument Systems, Sparks, MD)

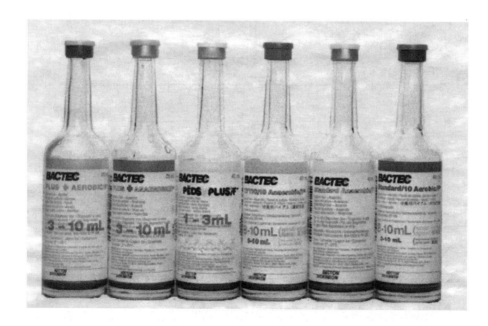

KNOWLEDGE LEVEL = 1

5. Which of the following anticoagulants is found in a royal blue-topped blood collection tube?
   A. lithium heparin
   B. no anticoagulant
   C. sodium citrate
   D. ammonium heparin

 KNOWLEDGE LEVEL = 1

6. The yellow-topped vacuum collection tube has which of the following additives?
   A. EDTA
   B. lithium heparin
   D. trisodium citrate
   C. sodium polyanetholesulfonate (SPS)

 KNOWLEDGE LEVEL = 2

7. Blood collection vacuum tubes may contain silicon to:
   A. decrease the possibility of hemolysis
   B. decrease interference between red blood cells and the anticoagulant
   C. create a barrier between the red blood cells and serum
   D. create a barrier between the red blood cells and plasma

 KNOWLEDGE LEVEL = 2

8. The blood collection set shown in Figure 7.2 is frequently used with the needle gauge size of:
   A. 21
   B. 19
   C. 18
   D. 17

FIGURE 7.2. Angel Wing blood collection set.

(Courtesy of Sherwood, Davis & Geck, St. Louis, MO)

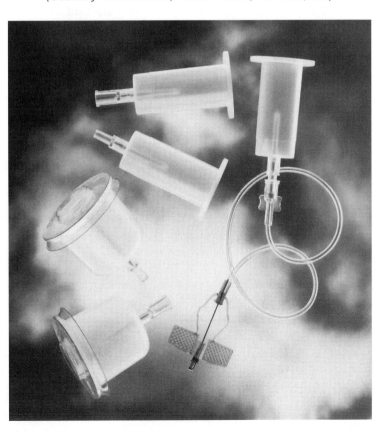

FIGURE 7.3.

(Courtesy of BD VACUTAINER Systems, Franklin Lakes, NJ)

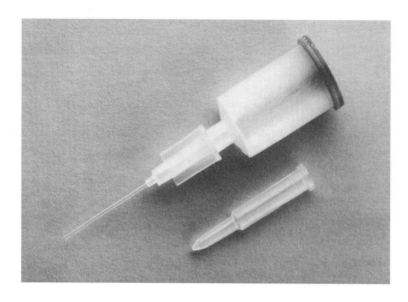

 KNOWLEDGE LEVEL = 2

9. For newborns, the penetration depth of lancets for blood collection must be:

A. 3.0 mm or less

B. 2.8 mm or less

C. 2.6 mm or less

D. 2.4 mm or less

 KNOWLEDGE LEVEL = 2

10. The blood collection device shown in Figure 7.3 can be used for:

A. microcollection of blood for sed rate

B. ABO group and type blood collection

C. microcollection and dilution of blood samples for the WBC count

D. microcollection of blood for culture and sensitivity testing

 KNOWLEDGE LEVEL = 2

11. Which of the following additives prevent coagulation of blood by removing calcium through the formation of insoluble calcium salts?

A. ammonium oxalate, EDTA, sodium heparin

B. EDTA, lithium heparin, sodium citrate

C. sodium fluoride, lithium heparin, EDTA

D. EDTA, sodium citrate, potassium oxalate

 KNOWLEDGE LEVEL = 1

12. Which of the listed needle gauges has the smallest diameter?

A. 19

B. 20

C. 21

D. 23

KNOWLEDGE LEVEL = 1

13. If the phlebotomist collects only venipuncture specimens, which of the following items would *not* be needed on his or her specimen collection tray?
    A. disposable gloves
    B. tourniquet
    C. alcohol, iodine, and Betadine pads
    D. Tenderletts (International Technidyne Corp., Edison, NJ)

 KNOWLEDGE LEVEL = 1

14. A blood cell count requires whole blood collected in a:
    A. green-topped tube
    B. purple-topped tube
    C. gray-topped tube
    D. light blue-topped tube

 KNOWLEDGE LEVEL = 2

15. The Autolet II Clinisafe (Owen Mumford, Inc.) is a:
    A. safety device for collecting arterial blood gas specimens
    B. safety device for collecting specimens by venipuncture
    C. safe method to dispose of sharps
    D. spring-activated puncture device for collecting capillary blood

 KNOWLEDGE LEVEL = 2

16. Specimens for which of the following tests must be collected in light blue-topped blood collection tubes?
    A. RVV time, Stypven time, APTT
    B. Stypven time, VDRL test, RPR test
    C. RPR test, PT, APTT
    D. Protime, Selenium, RVV test

 KNOWLEDGE LEVEL = 2

17. Which of the following tests usually requires blood collected in a royal blue-topped blood collection vacuum tube?
    A. cortisol level
    B. CBC level
    C. lactate dehydrogenase level
    D. lead level

 KNOWLEDGE LEVEL = 2

18. Which of the following is frequently used in the microcollection of electrolytes and general chemistry blood specimens?
    A. BD Unopette
    B. AVL Microsampler
    C. Helena Pumpette
    D. BD Microtainer

 KNOWLEDGE LEVEL = 1

19. Which of the following is a commonly used intravenous device that is sometimes used in the collection of blood from patients who are difficult to collect blood by conventional methods?
    A. heparinized Natelson tube
    B. BD Unopette
    C. butterfly needle
    D. BD Microtainer

 KNOWLEDGE LEVEL = 1

20. The assay for the enzyme alkaline phosphatase usually requires serum collected in a:
    A. green-topped tube
    B. purple-topped tube
    C. speckled-topped tube
    D. light blue-topped tube

KNOWLEDGE LEVEL = 1

21. Which of the following anticoagulants is found in a purple-topped blood collection vacuum tube?
A. EDTA
B. sodium heparin
C. ammonium oxalate
D. sodium oxalate

 KNOWLEDGE LEVEL = 1

22. Which of the following tests requires plasma collected in a purple-topped vacuum tube and transported in an ice water slurry?
A. bleeding-time test
B. leukocyte alkaline phosphatase
C. erythrocyte fragility test
D. renin activity test

 KNOWLEDGE LEVEL = 1

23. A prefilled device used as a collection and dilution unit is the:
A. BD Unopette
B. Monoject Corvac tube
C. heparinized Natelson tube
D. AVL microsampler

 KNOWLEDGE LEVEL = 1

24. Which of the following devices was developed specifically for the bleeding time assay?
A. Surgicutt
B. Autolet Lite Clinisafe
C. Tenderlett
D. Unopette

 KNOWLEDGE LEVEL = 1

25. The color coding for needles indicates the:
A. length
B. gauge
C. manufacturer
D. anticoagulant

 KNOWLEDGE LEVEL = 2

26. Which of the following blood analytes is sensitive to light?
A. lead
B. glucose
C. calcium
D. bilirubin

 KNOWLEDGE LEVEL = 1

27. Which of the following anticoagulants is used frequently in coagulation blood studies?
A. citrate-phosphate-dextrose (CPD)
B. potassium oxalate
C. acid-citrate-dextrose (ACD)
D. sodium citrate

 KNOWLEDGE LEVEL = 2

28. Which of the following is a serum separation tube?
A. heparinized Natelson tube
B. Hemalet
C. winged infusion set
D. Corvac tube

KNOWLEDGE LEVEL = 1

29. When blood is collected from a patient, the serum should be separated from the blood cells as quickly as possible to avoid:
    A. hemoconcentration
    B. hemolysis
    C. glycolysis
    D. hemostasis

 KNOWLEDGE LEVEL = 2

30. Blood collected for creatine kinase *cannot* be collected in a:
    A. red-topped tube
    B. gray-topped tube
    C. speckled-topped tube
    D. gold-topped tube

 KNOWLEDGE LEVEL = 1

31. Criteria used to describe vacuum collection tube size are:
    A. external tube diameter, maximum amount of specimen to be collected, and external tube length
    B. external tube diameter, minimum amount of specimen that can be collected, and external tube length
    C. internal tube diameter, maximum amount of specimen to be collected, and external tube length
    D. internal tube diameter, minimum amount of specimen that can be collected, and internal tube length

 KNOWLEDGE LEVEL = 1

32. The evacuated tube system requires:
    A. a special plastic adapter, a syringe, and an evacuated sample tube
    B. an evacuated sample tube, a plastic adapter, and a double-pointed needle

    C. a double-pointed needle, a plastic holder, and a winged infusion set
    D. a special plastic adapter, an anticoagulant, and a double-pointed needle

 KNOWLEDGE LEVEL = 3

33. The phlebotomist traveled to the home of 85-year-old Mrs. Ruth Harrison to collect blood for the PT, APTT, and potassium levels. Even though the blood collection was performed by using a winged infusion set on Mrs. Harrison's fragile veins, the light blue-topped tube was underfilled. However, the required amount of blood was collected in the green-topped tube. Which of the following will most likely occur?
    A. The potassium value will be falsely elevated.
    B. The PT and PTT results will be falsely prolonged.
    C. The potassium value will be falsely decreased.
    D. The PT and PTT results will not be affected.

 KNOWLEDGE LEVEL = 1

34. Blood for catecholamine levels needs to be collected in a:
    A. light blue-topped tube
    B. purple-topped tube
    C. speckled-topped tube
    D. green-topped tube

 KNOWLEDGE LEVEL = 1

35. Measurement of blood copper requires blood collection in a:
    A. light blue-topped tube
    B. green-topped tube
    C. royal blue-topped tube
    D. purple-topped tube

FIGURE 7.4.

(Courtesy of BD VACUTAINER Systems, Franklin Lakes, NJ)

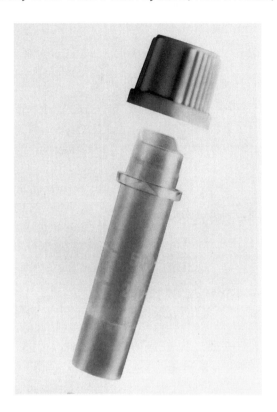

 KNOWLEDGE LEVEL = 1

36. Which of the following is frequently used for the microcollection of specimens for blood gas analysis?
    A. BD Unopette
    B. heparinized Natelson tubes
    C. BD Microtainer
    D. Autolet Lite Clinisafe

 KNOWLEDGE LEVEL = 1

37. The item in Figure 7.4 is usually referred to as a:
    A. Samplette capillary blood collector
    B. BD Microtainer
    C. Safe-T-Fill Capillary Blood Collection Device
    D. BD Unopette

 KNOWLEDGE LEVEL = 1

38. Which of the following anticoagulants is found in a green-topped blood collection vacuum tube?
    A. EDTA
    B. sodium heparin
    C. sodium citrate
    D. potassium oxalate

 KNOWLEDGE LEVEL = 2

39. Which of the following anticoagulants allows preparation of blood films with minimal distortion of WBCs?
    A. lithium heparin
    B. sodium citrate
    C. EDTA
    D. sodium heparin

KNOWLEDGE LEVEL = 1

40. The anticoagulant lithium heparin is most appropriate for blood collection to perform:
    A. measurement of sodium levels
    B. blood cell count, differential
    C. measurement of lithium levels
    D. PT and APTT

 KNOWLEDGE LEVEL = 1

41. The term A/G ratio refers to:
    A. alpha-antitrypsin/gamma glutamyl transpeptidase
    B. alpha-fibrinogen/globulin
    C. albumin/globulin
    D. albumin/gamma glutamyl transpeptidase

 KNOWLEDGE LEVEL = 1

42. Which of the following is an anticoagulant used in blood donations?
    A. sodium citrate
    B. citrate-phosphate-dextrose
    C. ethylene-diamine tetra-acetic acid
    D. lithium iodoacetate

 KNOWLEDGE LEVEL = 1

43. Which of the following contains an antiglycolytic agent?
    A. light blue-topped tube
    B. purple-topped tube
    C. gray-topped tube
    D. green-topped tube

 KNOWLEDGE LEVEL = 2

44. Antidiuretic hormone (ADH) requires which of the following blood collection tubes for proper test results?
    A. speckled-topped tube
    B. light blue-topped tube
    C. royal blue-topped tube
    D. purple-topped tube

 KNOWLEDGE LEVEL = 3

45. Which of the following procedures requires the patient to be recumbent for at least 30 minutes before blood collection?
    A. alkaline phosphatase
    B. aldosterone
    C. adrenocorticotropic hormone
    D. acetaminophen

 KNOWLEDGE LEVEL = 1

46. Which of the following should be collected in a royal blue-topped tube?
    A. phenobarbital
    B. nickel
    C. procainamide
    D. 5′ nucleotidase

 KNOWLEDGE LEVEL = 2

47. The enzyme aspartate aminotransferase is sometimes listed on the laboratory request form as:
    A. SGOT
    B. SGPT
    C. ALT
    D. ALP

KNOWLEDGE LEVEL = 2

48. John, a phlebotomist who collects only capillary blood from patients in the newborn and pediatric units, probably would have all of the following equipment on his blood collection tray except:
   A. BD Unopettes
   B. sterile gauze pads
   C. serum separator BD VACUTAINER tubes
   D. biohazardous waste container for sharps

 KNOWLEDGE LEVEL = 2

49. The volume of plasma or serum that generally can be collected from a premature infant is approximately:
   A. 50 to 100 mL
   B. 100 to 150 mL
   C. 150 to 200 mL
   D. 250 to 300 mL

 KNOWLEDGE LEVEL = 1

50. The red and green speckled-topped blood collection tube should be gently inverted five times so that blood clotting occurs in:
   A. 5 minutes
   B. 15 minutes
   C. 30 minutes
   D. 45 minutes

 KNOWLEDGE LEVEL = 2

51. To avoid microclotting in the blood collection tube, it is extremely important that the blood collected in a purple-topped tube be gently inverted a minimum of:
   A. 0 times
   B. 5 times
   C. 8 times
   D. 12 times

 KNOWLEDGE LEVEL = 1

52. The glucose-6-phosphate dehydrogenase quantitative procedure requires blood to be collected in a:
   A. gray-topped tube
   B. green-topped tube
   C. red-topped tube
   D. light blue-topped tube

 KNOWLEDGE LEVEL = 2

53. The physician requested that a creatine kinase procedure be performed STAT on Mrs. Billingsworth in Room 4220. The phlebotomist needs to collect the blood required for the procedure in a:
   A. red and green speckled-topped tube
   B. light blue-topped tube
   C. gray-topped tube
   D. yellow and green speckled-topped tube

 KNOWLEDGE LEVEL = 1

54. Which of the following tests requires blood to be collected in a red-topped tube?
   A. cortisol
   B. Coombs' test
   C. cryofibrinogen
   D. chromium

 KNOWLEDGE LEVEL = 1

55. The highest percentage of needle stick injuries has been shown to occur using the:
   A. 22-gauge needle with the evacuated tube system
   B. syringe needle
   C. S-Monovette
   D. winged infusion sets

KNOWLEDGE LEVEL = 1

56. The cardiac troponins assay needs to have a blood specimen collected in a:
    A. green-topped tube
    B. speckled-topped tube
    C. light blue-topped tube
    D. purple-topped tube

 KNOWLEDGE LEVEL = 1

57. The blood collection for phenylalanine testing requires a:
    A. light blue-topped tube
    B. blood smear
    C. special filter paper
    D. purple-topped tube

 KNOWLEDGE LEVEL = 1

58. ESR is the same laboratory assay as:
    A. estradiol
    B. sed rate
    C. E-rosette receptor
    D. ethosuximide

 KNOWLEDGE LEVEL = 1

59. T_4 is the same laboratory assay as:
    A. thyroxine
    B. thyroglobulin
    C. triiodothyronine
    D. thyroid antibodies

 KNOWLEDGE LEVEL = 1

60. If blood needs to be collected for syphilis testing, which of the following tests should the phlebotomist collect blood for?
    A. RPR
    B. TSH
    C. RVV
    D. *Proteus* OX 19

 KNOWLEDGE LEVEL = 2

61. Blood collected for electrolytes is used to measure:
    A. Ni, K, Cl
    B. Na, K, Cu
    C. Na, K, Cl
    D. Na, Se, Cl

 KNOWLEDGE LEVEL = 1

62. Which of the following is the best for the sterile blood collection of trace elements, toxicology, and nutritional studies?
    A. gold-topped tube
    B. royal blue-topped tube
    C. purple-topped tube
    D. yellow-topped tube

 KNOWLEDGE LEVEL = 1

63. To collect for blood ammonia levels, which of the following blood collection tubes is required?
    A. green-topped tube
    B. purple-topped tube
    C. red and yellow speckled-topped tube
    D. royal blue-topped tube

KNOWLEDGE LEVEL = 1

64. Which of the following analytes needs to be collected in a royal blue-topped blood collection tube?

    A. potassium
    B. magnesium
    C. manganese
    D. methotrexate

 KNOWLEDGE LEVEL = 2

65. Which of the following blood analytes does *not* have to have the collected blood transported in an ice slurry?

    A. insulin
    B. renin activity
    C. lactic acid
    D. lactate dehydrogenase

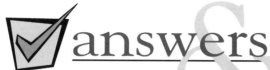

answers & rationales

1.

A. The Microtome is a cutting device used in histology.

B. The S-Monovette (Sarstedt, Inc., Newton, NC) is used for venipuncture collections.

C. The Safety-Gard Phlebotomy System (BD VACUTAINER Systems, Franklin Lakes, NJ) is used for venipuncture collection.

D. The Samplette capillary blood collector (Sherwood, Davis & Geck, St. Louis, MO) is offered with a full range of additives for capillary blood collection. (p. 216)

2.

A. Chromosome analysis requires whole blood collected in a green-topped (Na heparin) blood collection tube. (p. 89)

B. Red-topped tubes contain no additive, but sodium heparin is required for chromosome analysis.

C. Gray-topped tubes contain potassium oxalate and sodium fluoride or lithium iodoacetate and heparin, which will interfere in chromosome analysis.

D. Light blue-topped tubes contain sodium citrate, which will interfere in chromosome analysis.

3.

A. Microscopy specimens are usually urine collections and therefore do not require a blood collection system.

B. Clinical chemistry specimens do not require culture media vials as shown in Figure 7.1.

C. Clinical immunology specimens do not require culture media vials as shown in Figure 7.1.

D. The BACTEC culture vials shown in Figure 7.1 (courtesy of Becton-Dickinson Diagnostic Instrument Systems, Sparks, MD) are used for microbiology blood collections. (p. 199)

4.

A. The erythrocyte sedimentation rate requires a black-topped tube with sodium citrate or purple-topped tubes with EDTA.

B. Zinc levels may be erroneous if collected with lithium heparin, since the green-topped tubes are not manufactured for trace element collections.

C. Lithium heparin is found in green-topped tubes and is very suitable for blood glucose measurements. (p. 198)

D. The blood lithium level will be falsely increased if collected with lithium heparin anticoagulant.

5.

A. Lithium heparin is generally found in green-topped tubes, not royal blue.

B. Royal blue-topped tubes generally contain sodium heparin, EDTA, or no anticoagulant. (p. 180)

C. Sodium citrate is generally used in light blue-topped tubes.

D. Ammonium heparin is not used generally in blood collection tubes.

6.

A. EDTA is used in purple-topped collection tubes.

B. Lithium heparin is generally used in green-topped tubes.

C. Trisodium citrate is normally used in light blue-topped tubes.

D. Sodium polyanetholesulfonate (SPS) is used in the collection of blood culture specimens. (pp. 198–199, 338)

7.

A. Silicon is used in the collection tubes to decrease the possibility of hemolysis. (p. 178)

B. The silicon does not react with the anticoagulant but rather works as a lubricant in the collection tube.

C. A polymer barrier, not silicon, is used to create a barrier between the red blood cells and serum.

D. A polymer barrier, not silicon, is used to create a barrier between the red blood cells and plasma.

8.

A. The needle sizes of 21, 23, and 25 gauge are generally used with the blood collection set (courtesy of Sherwood, Davis & Geck, Inc, St. Louis, MO). (p. 201)

B. The needle size of 19 gauge is generally not used with a blood collection set, since it has a large interior bore.

C. The needle size of 18 gauge is generally not used with a blood collection set, since it has a large interior bore.

D. The needle size of 17 gauge is generally not used with a blood collection set, since it has a large interior bore.

9.

A. A depth of 3.0 mm can possibly penetrate the bone in a newborn.

B. A depth of 2.8 mm can possibly penetrate the bone in a newborn.

C. A depth of 2.6 mm can possibly penetrate the bone in a newborn.

D. For newborns, lancets with tips 2.4 mm or less in length are required to avoid penetrating bone. (p. 211)

10.

A. The sed rate procedure requires undiluted whole blood, and therefore, the Unopette—a collection and dilution unit—cannot be used.

B. ABO group and type blood procedure requires whole blood or serum, and therefore the diluting fluid in the Unopette cannot be used.

C. The Unopette shown in Figure 7.3 (courtesy of BD VACUTAINER Systems, Franklin Lakes, NJ) is a collection and dilution unit used for various procedures, including the WBC count, RBC count, platelet count, hemoglobin, RBC fragility, and sodium, potassium, and lead determinations. (p. 219)

D. Blood collection for blood cultures requires at least 3 mL of whole blood collected in culture vials or SPS tubes, not in a microcollection and dilution Unopette vial.

11.

A. Ammonium oxalate and EDTA prevent coagulation of blood by removing calcium and forming insoluble calcium salts. However, heparin prevents coagulation by inactivating blood-clotting thrombin and thromboplastin.

B. EDTA and sodium citrate prevent blood coagulation by removing calcium through the formation of insoluble calcium salts. However, lithium heparin prevents blood clotting by inactivating thrombin and thromboplastin.

C. Sodium fluoride is an additive to inhibit glycolytic action (glucose breakdown). Lithium heparin prevents coagulation by inactivating blood clotting thrombin and thromboplastin. EDTA does prevent blood coagulation through the formation of insoluble calcium salts.

D. Coagulation of blood can be prevented by the addition of oxalates, citrates, and/or EDTA by their ability to remove calcium, forming insoluble calcium salts. (p. 185)

12.

A. The smaller the gauge number, the larger the diameter of the needle.

B. The smaller the gauge number, the larger the diameter of the needle.

C. The smaller the gauge number, the larger the diameter of the needle.

D. The smaller the gauge number, the larger the diameter of the needle. (p. 201)

13.

A. Disposable gloves need to be worn for any kind of blood collection.

B. The tourniquet is needed to slow down venous flow for venipuncture.

C. Alcohol, iodine, and Betadine pads are cleansing agents that are needed in venipuncture to cleanse the blood collection site.

D. Tenderletts (International Technidyne Corp., Edison, NJ) are safety, single-use, automatically retracting, disposable devices used for microcollection by skin puncture. (p. 212)

14.

A. Green-topped tubes contain heparin that can alter the accuracy of blood cell counts.

B. A blood cell count, including WBC count, RBC count, hemoglobin (Hgb), hematocrit (Hct), mean corpuscular volume (MCV), mean corpuscular hemoglobin (MCH), and mean corpuscular hemoglobin concentration (MCHC), requires whole blood collected in a purple-topped blood collection tube. (pp. 187–188)

C. Gray-topped tubes contain sodium fluoride and potassium oxalate or lithium iodoacetate and heparin. These additives can falsely alter the blood cell count levels.

D. Light blue-topped tubes contain sodium citrate and will alter the accuracy of the blood cell count levels.

15.

A. The Autolet II Clinisafe is a safety device for skin puncture rather than arterial puncture.

B. The Autolet II Clinisafe is a safety device for skin puncture rather than venipuncture.

C. The Autolet II Clinisafe is a safety device for skin puncture with an enclosed lancet. Therefore it is not for disposal of sharps.

D. The Autolet II Clinisafe is a spring-activated puncture device with three disposable platforms for control and penetration depth. (p. 212)

16.

A. Stypven time, also known as RVV time and APTT (activated partial thromboplastin time), are laboratory tests requiring blood collection in the light blue-topped tubes containing citrate. (pp. 187, 195, 197)

B. Stypven time is a coagulation procedure requiring collection in a light blue-topped tube. The VDRL and RPR tests are syphilis tests requiring serum collected in red- or speckled-topped tubes.

C. The RPR test is used to detect syphilis in blood and requires a red- or speckled-topped tube for collection.

PT and APTT tests are coagulation procedures that are run on blood collected in the light blue-topped tubes.

D. Protime (PT) and RVV test are coagulation procedures that are performed on blood collected in the light blue-topped tube. However, selenium (Se) is a trace element and must be tested on blood collected in a trace element tube (royal blue-topped with heparin) or in EDTA (purple-topped tube).

17.

A. Cortisol is a hormone, and to measure it, blood needs to be collected in a green-topped tube.

B. CBC level requires blood collected in EDTA—a purple-topped tube.

C. The enzyme, lactate dehydrogenase, needs to be detected in a blood sample collected with a speckled-topped tube.

D. Lead levels in blood are very minute and require a blood collection tube without any detectable lead such as the royal blue-topped tube. (p. 193)

18.

A. The BD Unopette can be used for blood measurements of sodium and potassium. However, this device is not used for general chemistry blood sampling.

B. The AVL microsampler is used for the collection of arterial blood required for blood gas analysis.

C. The Helena Pumpette is a device that can provide access to the needed blood sample without uncapping the blood collection tube. It is not a microcollection device.

D. The BD Microtainer tube is frequently used in the microcollection of electrolytes and general chemistry blood specimens. (pp. 216–217)

19.

A. Heparinized Natelson tubes are used for microcollection of blood rather than an intravenous device.

B. The BD Unopette is a microcollection and dilution device that is used to measure various analytes.

C. The butterfly needle, also referred to as winged infusion set, is the most commonly used intravenous device. (p. 201)

D. The BD Microtainer is a microcollection device that is used to collect blood from a skin puncture site.

20.

A. The green-topped tube contains heparin, which could possibly interfere in the measurement of the enzyme alkaline phosphatase.

B. The purple-topped tube contains the anticoagulant EDTA, which can interfere in the measurement of alkaline phosphatase.

C. The speckled-topped tube contains a serum separator barrier but no anticoagulants and therefore is appropriate for measurement of the enzyme alkaline phosphatase. (p. 186)

D. The light blue-topped tube contains citrate, which can interfere in the measurement of the enzyme alkaline phosphatase.

21.

A. The anticoagulant EDTA is found in a purple-topped blood collection vacuum tube. (p. 198)

B. Sodium heparin is the anticoagulant used in green-topped blood collection vacuum tubes.

C. Ammonium oxalate is an anticoagulant that was used in the past but has been replaced by other additives.

D. Sodium oxalate is currently not used as an anticoagulant and is therefore not in the purple-topped vacuum tube.

22.

A. The bleeding-time test does not require collection in a vacuum tube or transportation in an ice water slurry.

B. The leukocyte alkaline phosphatase measurement requires six fresh blood smears.

C. The erythrocyte fragility test requires whole blood collected in a purple-topped tube *without* transportation in an ice water slurry.

D. Renin activity level is a fragile blood analyte that must be collected in the EDTA-containing purple-topped vacuum tube and transported in an ice water slurry. (p. 195)

23.

A. The BD Unopette is a blood collection device that is prefilled with specific amounts of diluents or reagents. (p. 219)

B. The Sherwood, Davis & Geck, Inc. Monoject Corvac Serum Separator tube is used for venipuncture collections and does not have a dilution unit.

C. Heparinized Natelson tubes are capillary tubes for microcollection but are not prefilled with a solution for dilution of the blood.

D. AVL microsampler is a special syringe for arterial blood sample collections.

24.

A. Surgicutt is a sterile, standardized, disposable instrument that is used for bleeding time assay. (p. 331)

B. The Autolet Lite Clinisafe is a safety microcollection device.

C. The Tenderlett is a safety microcollection device.

D. The BD Unopette is a blood collection and dilution device used in the measurement of the RBC count, WBC count, platelet count, and other procedures but not bleeding time.

25.

A. The length of the needle is *not* indicated by a color code. The gauge of the needle is indicated by the color code.

B. The gauge size of the needle is identified by the color code on the sealed shield. (p. 201)

C. The color code on the shield indicates the gauge of the needle, not the manufacturer.

D. The blood collection tubes contain additives as shown by their tops. Needles have color-coded shields to indicate gauge size.

26.

A. Lead is an analyte that must be collected in a royal blue-topped vacuum tube, but it does not have to be protected from light.

B. Glucose is not chemically degraded when exposed to light, and therefore blood for glucose measurement does not require protection from light.

C. Calcium is not chemically degraded when exposed to light, and therefore blood collected for calcium determinations does not need to be protected from light.

D. Bilirubin breaks down chemically when exposed to light, and thus, the blood must be protected from light when bilirubin is to be measured. (p. 187)

27.

A. Citrate-phosphate-dextrose (CPD) is an anticoagulant and preservative that is frequently used in the collection of blood for blood donations.

B. Potassium oxalate is an anticoagulant that is used in the gray-topped vacuum tubes for blood glucose testing.

C. Acid-citrate-dextrose (ACD) is an anticoagulant and preservative that is frequently used in the collection of blood for blood donation.

D. Sodium citrate, the anticoagulant in light blue-topped blood collection tubes, is frequently used in coagulation blood studies. (p. 198)

28.

A. The heparinized Natelson tube is a microcollection capillary tube that contains heparin to mix with the blood to avoid blood coagulation.

B. Hemalet (Medprobe Laboratories, New York, NY) is an automatic blade-retraction device for the bleeding time test.

C. The winged infusion set is a stainless steel beveled needle and tube with attached plastic wings.

D. The Corvac tube (Sherwood, Davis & Geck, Inc.) contains a gel with a specific gravity intermediate to serum and coagulum, forming a stable barrier between serum and coagulum. (p. 199)

29.

A. Hemoconcentration sometimes occurs in the patient at the venipuncture site because of several factors, including prolonged tourniquet application, squeezing and probing the site.

B. Hemolysis is the breakdown of RBCs, which is not the most critical reason for separating blood cells from the serum.

C. Glycolysis is the breakdown of glucose, which can lead to erroneously low blood glucose results if the red blood cells are not separated from the serum. (p. 185)

D. Hemostasis is the maintenance of circulating blood in the liquid state and retention of blood in the vascular system within the human body.

30.

A. Blood for creatine kinase can be collected in the red-topped tube, since it contains no interfering additives.

B. The gray-topped tube contains fluoride, which will break down the enzyme creatine kinase and give a falsely low level. (p. 198)

C. Blood for creatine kinase can be collected in the speckled-topped tube, since it separates serum from blood cells and has no affect on the creatine kinase level.

D. Blood for creatine kinase can be collected in the gold-topped tube, since it contains no interfering additives.

31.

A. The external tube diameter and length plus the maximum amount of specimen to be collected into the vacuum tube are the criteria that are used to describe vacuum collection tube size. (p. 179)

B. Two criteria are correct: the external tube diameter and length. However, it is the maximum rather than minimum amount of specimen that can be collected as the third criterion.

C. Maximum amount of specimen to be collected and external tube length are two correct criteria. However, the third criterion is external rather than internal tube diameter.

D. All three criteria are incorrect for this distracter. The correct criteria should be external rather than internal tube diameter and tube length. Also, the third criterion should be the maximum rather than minimum amount of specimen to be collected.

32.

A. A syringe is not part of the evacuated tube system; the plastic adapter, evacuated sample tube, and double-pointed needle are the three parts of the system.

B. The evacuated tube system requires three components: the evacuated sample tube, the double-pointed needle, and a special plastic adapter. (p. 178)

C. The double-pointed needle and plastic holder are two parts of the evacuated tube system. However, the winged infusion set, also referred to as the butterfly, is not considered the third part of the evacuated tube system.

D. A special plastic adapter and double-pointed needle are two parts of the evacuated tube system; the third component is the evacuated sample tube rather than anticoagulant.

33.

A. The potassium value is determined from the blood collected in the green-topped tube. Since the required amount of blood was collected in this tube, the result should not be erroneously affected.

B. If a light blue-topped tube is underfilled, coagulation results will be erroneously prolonged. (p. 198)

C. The potassium value is determined from the blood collected in the green-topped tube. Since the required amount of blood was collected in this tube, the result should not be erroneously affected.

D. The PT and PTT tests are performed on blood collected with the anticoagulant sodium citrate. If the required blood level is not collected in the sodium citrate tube, then the ratio of sodium citrate to blood is increased, causing erroneously prolonged coagulation results.

34.

A. The light blue-topped tube contains citrate, which is not the appropriate anticoagulant for collection of catecholamines.

B. The blood for catecholamine levels needs to be collected in a purple-topped tube and transported in an ice water slurry. (p. 188)

C. The speckled-topped tube contains a gel barrier for separation of serum from red blood cells. However, blood catecholamine levels require measurement on whole blood.

D. The green-topped tube contains heparin, which is not the appropriate anticoagulant for collection of catecholamines.

35.

A. The light blue-topped tube contains citrate and is usually used for collection of blood for coagulation procedures.

B. The green-topped tube contains the anticoagulant heparin and is usually used for chemistry tests, but not trace element testing.

C. The royal blue-topped tube is designed for collection of trace elements such as copper. (pp. 189, 198)

D. The purple-topped tube contains the anticoagulant EDTA and is generally used for hematology testing.

36.

A. The BD Unopette is a microcollection device that serves as a collection and dilution unit for the measurement of several analytes, including WBC count, RBC count, platelet count, and hemoglobin.

B. The Natelson collecting tubes (pipettes) are used with lithium heparin to collect blood for blood gas analysis. (p. 215)

C. The BD Microtainer is a microcollection tube that is used for blood collection to measure several chemistry analytes but not blood gas analysis.

D. The Autolet Lite Clinisafe is a spring-activated puncture device for skin puncture.

37.

A. The Samplette capillary blood collection device (Sherwood, Davis & Geck, St. Louis, MO) is not shown in Figure 7.4, but it is also a blood microcollection device.

B. The BD Microtainer (BD VACUTAINER Systems, Franklin Lakes, NJ) is shown in Figure 7.4 and is used frequently for electrolytes and general chemistry microspecimens. (pp. 216–217)

C. The Safe-T-Fill Capillary Blood Collection device (RAM Scientific Co., Needham, MA) is not shown in Figure 7.4, but it is also used in the microcollection of blood for various analytes.

D. The BD Unopette (BD VACUTAINER Systems, Franklin Lakes, NJ) is not shown in Figure 7.4; it is a type of device that serves as a collection and dilution unit for blood samples.

38.

A. The anticoagulant EDTA is found in a purple-topped blood collection vacuum tube.

B. The anticoagulant sodium heparin is found in a green-topped blood collection vacuum tube. (p. 198)

C. The anticoagulant sodium citrate is found in a light blue-topped blood collection vacuum tube.

D. The anticoagulant potassium oxalate is found in a gray-topped blood collection vacuum tube.

39.

A. Lithium heparin is not suitable for blood smears because the anticoagulant interferes in the staining process.

B. Sodium citrate is generally not used in the preparation of blood smears, since it can create alterations in the staining process.

C. Ethylene-diamine tetra-acetic acid (EDTA) is used to collect blood for blood smears, since it creates minimal distortion of WBCs. (p. 185)

D. Sodium heparin is not suitable for blood smears because the anticoagulant interferes in the staining process.

40.

A. The anticoagulant lithium heparin is very appropriate for blood collection to measure sodium and other chemistry analytes, except lithium levels. (p. 198)

B. Lithium heparin should not be used for collection for blood smears because the heparin causes the Wright's stain to have a blue background.

C. The anticoagulant lithium heparin should not be used to collect blood for the measurement of lithium levels, since it will lead to a falsely elevated level.

D. PT and APTT are coagulation procedures that need blood collected with the anticoagulant sodium citrate.

41.

A. Alpha-antitrypsin and gamma glutamyl transpeptidase are completely different assays.

B. Alpha-fibrinogen is not actually a laboratory assay, but globulin is tested with albumin as a ratio.

C. The term A/G refers to albumin/globulin ratio. (p. 197)

D. Albumin is tested with globulin as a ratio rather than the enzyme gamma glutamyl transpeptidase.

42.

A. Sodium citrate is an anticoagulant that is used generally for collection of blood to test for coagulation abnormalities.

B. Citrate-phosphate-dextrose (CPD) is one of the anticoagulants that is used extensively in blood donations. (p. 185)

C. Ethylene-diamine tetra-acetic acid (EDTA) is the anticoagulant found in the purple-topped tube for hematology testing.

D. Lithium iodoacetate is the anticoagulant found in the gray-topped tube for glucose testing.

43.

A. The light blue-topped tube contains sodium citrate, which is an anticoagulant but not an antiglycolytic agent.

B. The purple-topped tube contains EDTA, which is an anticoagulant but not an antiglycolytic agent.

C. The gray-topped tube contains sodium fluoride or lithium iodoacetate, which are antiglycolytic agents. (p. 185)

D. The green-topped tube contains lithium or sodium heparin, which is an anticoagulant but not an antiglycolytic agent.

44.

A. Antidiuretic hormone (ADH) testing requires a whole blood sample collected in a purple-topped tube. The speckled-topped tube separates blood cells from serum.

B. Antidiuretic hormone (ADH) testing requires a whole blood sample collected in a purple-topped tube.

C. Antidiuretic hormone (ADH) testing requires a whole blood sample collected in a purple-topped tube.

D. Antidiuretic hormone (ADH) testing requires blood collected in a purple-topped tube. (p. 187)

45.

A. Alkaline phosphatase does not require the patient to be recumbent for at least 30 minutes before blood collection but requires only a blood sample collected in a speckled-topped tube.

B. Aldosterone testing requires the patient to be recumbent for at least 30 minutes before blood collection. (p. 186)

C. Adrenocorticotropic hormone (ACTH) requires only a whole blood sample collected in a purple-topped tube. The patient has no restrictions before the blood collection.

D. Acetaminophen (Tylenol) does not require the patient to be recumbent for at least 30 minutes before blood collection but requires only a blood sample collected in a speckled-topped tube.

46.

A. The blood for the phenobarbital needs to be collected in a speckled-topped tube.

B. Nickel (Ni) is a trace element and therefore should be collected in the royal blue-topped tube designed for collection of trace elements. (p. 194)

C. The blood for procainamide testing needs to be collected in a speckled-topped tube.

D. The blood for 5′ nucleotidase needs to be collected in a speckled-topped tube.

47.

A. The enzyme aspartate aminotransferase is sometimes listed on the laboratory request form as SGOT. (p. 195)

B. SGPT is also listed as alanine aminotransferase or ALT.

C. ALT is also listed as alanine aminotransferase or SGPT.

D. ALP is also listed as alkaline phosphatase.

48.

A. Unopettes are blood collection and dilution devices used in microcollection for various assays.

B. Sterile gauze pads are required in both venipuncture and skin puncture.

C. Serum separator BD VACUTAINER tubes are used for venipuncture collections rather than microcollections. Since microcollection is the procedure used by the phlebotomist, he uses microcollection tubes rather than BD VACUTAINERS. (p. 220)

D. Biohazard waste containers for sharps are used for venipuncture and skin puncture procedures.

49.

A. The volume of plasma or serum that generally can be collected from a premature infant is approximately 100 to 150 mL.

B. The volume of plasma or serum that generally can be collected from a premature infant is approximately 100 to 150 mL. (p. 211)

C. The volume of plasma or serum that generally can be collected from a premature infant is approximately 100 to 150 mL.

D. The volume of plasma or serum that generally can be collected from a premature infant is approximately 100 to 150 mL.

50.

A. The red and green speckled-topped blood collection tube should be gently inverted five times so that blood clotting occurs in 30 minutes.

B. The red and green speckled-topped blood collection tube should be gently inverted five times so that blood clotting occurs in 30 minutes.

C. The red and green speckled-topped blood collection tube should be gently inverted five times so that blood clotting occurs in 30 minutes. (in the back of the *Phlebotomy Handbook*)

D. The red and green speckled-topped blood collection tube should be gently inverted five times so that blood clotting occurs in 30 minutes.

51.

A. The purple-topped tube must be gently inverted at least eight times after blood collection to prevent clotting.

B. The purple-topped tube must be gently inverted at least eight times after blood collection to prevent clotting.

C. The purple-topped tube must be gently inverted at least eight times after blood collection to prevent clotting. (in the back of the *Phlebotomy Handbook*)

D. The purple-topped tube must be gently inverted at least eight times after blood collection to prevent clotting.

52.

A. Glucose-6-phosphate dehydrogenase quantitative procedure requires blood to be collected in a green-topped tube.

B. Glucose-6-phosphate dehydrogenase quantitative procedure requires blood to be collected in a green-topped tube. (p. 191)

C. Glucose-6-phosphate dehydrogenase quantitative procedure requires blood to be collected in a green-topped tube.

D. Glucose-6-phosphate dehydrogenase quantitative procedure requires blood to be collected in a green-topped tube.

53.

A. Creatine kinase testing requires serum. The red and green speckled-topped tube yields blood cells and serum, but it requires at least 30 minutes for blood clotting.

B. Creatine kinase testing requires serum, whereas blood collected in the light blue-topped tube yields blood cells and plasma.

C. Gray-topped tubes contain fluoride, which destroys the blood enzymes (i.e., creatine kinase).

D. For STAT serum determinations in chemistry (e.g., creatine kinase), the yellow and green speckled-topped tube ensures complete clotting usually in less than 5 minutes. (in the back of the *Phlebotomy Handbook*)

54.

A. Cortisol testing requires that blood be collected in a green-topped tube.

B. The Coombs' test requires a blood specimen collected in a red-topped tube. (p. 189)

C. Cryofibrinogen testing requires that blood be collected in a green-topped tube.

D. Chromium testing requires that blood be collected in a royal blue-topped tube.

55.

A. The 22-gauge needle with an unguarded adapter needle aparatus can lead to needle stick injuries, but the winged-infusion sets account for the highest percentage of needlestick injuries.

B. The syringe with an unguarded needle can lead to needlestick injuries, but the winged-infusion sets account for the highest percentage of needle stick injuries.

C. The S-Monovette (Sarsedt, Inc., Newton, NC) is a safety device for vacuum collection or the syringe collection technique. It is designed to eliminate needlestick injuries.

D. Winged-infusion sets also referred to as blood collection sets or the butterfly needle, have been shown to account for the highest percentage of needlestick injuries. (p. 201)

56.

A. The green-topped tube is used for several chemistry assay collections, but the cardiac troponins assay requires a blood specimen collected in a speckled-topped tube.

B. The cardiac troponins assay requires a blood specimen collected in a speckled-topped tube. (p. 188)

C. The light blue-topped-tube is generally used for collection of blood for coagulation assays, not the cardiac troponins assay.

D. The purple-topped tube is generally used for collection of blood for hematology assays, not the cardiac troponins chemistry assays.

57.

A. Phenylalanine blood testing requires blood collected on a special filter paper rather than in a vacuum collection tube.

B. Phenylalanine blood testing requires blood collected on a special filter paper rather than a blood smear.

C. Phenylalanine testing requires that blood droplets should be collected on filter paper with a low background fluorescence. (p. 194)

D. Phenylalanine blood testing requires blood collected on a special filter paper rather than in a vacuum collection tube.

58.

A. ESR is the same laboratory assay as a sedimentation rate, erythrocyte sedimentation rate, or sed rate.

B. ESR is the same laboratory assay as a sedimentation rate, erythrocyte sedimentation rate, or sed rate. (p. 190)

C. ESR is the same laboratory assay as a sedimentation rate, erythrocyte sedimentation rate, or sed rate.

D. ESR is the same laboratory assay as a sedimentation rate, erythrocyte sedimentation rate, or sed rate.

59.

A. T_4 is also referred to as thyroxine. (p. 196)

B. Thyroglobulin is a thyroid assay, but it is not referred to as T_4. T_4 is thyroxine.

C. Triiodothyronine is the same laboratory assay as T_3.

D. Thyroid antibodies are not the same as T_4. T_4 refers to thyroxine.

60.

A. Rapid plasma reagin (RPR) is the syphilis assay that needs the blood collected in a speckled-topped tube. (p. 197)

B. TSH is the same as thyrotropin or thyroid-stimulating hormone. It is a test for thyroid function.

C. RVV is the abbreviation for Russell Viper Venom time, a blood coagulation procedure.

D. *Proteus* OX 19 is a serology assay performed on blood collected in a speckled-topped tube.

61.

A. Sodium (Na), potassium (K), and chloride (Cl) are all important blood electrolytes. Nickel (Ni) is a trace element that has electrolytic activity but does not affect the other blood analytes and body organs as much as Na, K, and Cl.

B. Sodium (Na), potassium (K), and chloride (Cl) are all important blood electrolytes. Copper (Cu) is a trace element that has electrolytic activity but does not affect the other blood analytes and body organs as much as Na, K, and Cl.

C. Sodium (Na), potassium (K), and chloride (Cl) are all important blood electrolytes. (p. 190)

D. Sodium (Na) and chloride (Cl) are blood electrolytes, but selenium (Se) is a trace element.

62.

A. The gold-topped tube has a polymer barrier for the separation of clotted blood from serum and is used for general chemistry testing.

B. The royal blue-topped tube has been designed to collect sterile blood specimens for trace elements, toxicology, and/or nutritional studies. (p. 180)

C. The purple-topped tube contains the anticoagulant EDTA and is frequently used for hematology studies.

D. The yellow-topped tube contains sodium polyanetholesulfonate (SPS) for the collection of blood culture specimens.

63.

A. The green-topped tube contains heparin, a mucopolysaccharide that is used for ammonia blood collection. (p. 186)

B. The purple-topped tube contains the anticoagulant EDTA and is used for hematology studies, not ammonia levels.

C. The red and yellow speckled-topped tube contains a polymer barrier for the separation of the blood clot from serum. Blood ammonia levels require whole blood, and therefore the red and yellow speckled-topped tube is not appropriate.

D. The royal blue-topped tube is for the collection of trace elements, toxicology, and nutritional studies but not ammonia levels.

64.

A. Potassium is one of the major blood electrolytes and is not a trace element. Therefore potassium levels are collected in green-topped, speckled-topped, or red-topped tubes rather than royal blue-topped tubes.

B. Magnesium is collected in a speckled-topped tube, since it is not a trace element.

C. Manganese (Mn) is a trace element and needs to be tested by blood collected in the royal blue-topped tube. (p. 193)

D. Methotrexate is a medication that therapeutically is monitored in blood analysis using blood collected in a red-topped tube.

65.

A. Insulin analysis requires blood collected in a purple-topped tube and transported in an ice slurry.

B. Renin activity requires blood collected in a purple-topped tube and transported in an ice slurry.

C. Lactic acid analysis requires blood collected in a gray-topped tube and transported in an ice slurry.

D. Blood for lactate dehydrogenase does not require transportation in an ice slurry. (p. 193)

8 Venipuncture Procedures

chapter objectives

Upon completion of Chapter 8, the learner is responsible for the following:

➤ Describe the patient identification process for inpatients, emergency room patients, and ambulatory patients.

➤ List essential information for test requisitions.

➤ List supplies that would be used in a typical venipuncture procedure.

➤ Identify the most common sites for venipuncture, and describe situations in which these sites might not be acceptable sites for venipuncture. Identify alternative sites for the venipuncture procedure.

➤ Describe the process and the time limits for applying a tourniquet to a patient's arm.

➤ Describe the decontamination process and the agents that are used to decontaminate skin for routine blood tests and blood cultures.

➤ Describe the actual venipuncture procedure and the steps that are different using the evacuated tube method, the syringe method, and the butterfly or winged infusion system.

➤ Describe the order of draw for collection tubes when using the evacuated tube method, the syringe method, and the butterfly or winged infusion system.

➤ List examples and explain reasons for the importance of collecting timed specimens at the requested times.

➤ Describe the proper method for hand washing.

➤ Define the terms "fasting" and "STAT."

DIRECTIONS Each of the questions or incomplete statements below is followed by four suggested answers or completions. Select **one answer** that is best in each case.

 KNOWLEDGE LEVEL = 1

1. Identification of an inpatient can best be accomplished by which of the following?
   A. number on the hospital bracelet and verbal confirmation from the patient
   B. hospital room number and bed assignment
   C. confirmation from a patient's relative
   D. none of the above

 KNOWLEDGE LEVEL = 1

2. Information on an inpatient's identification bracelet usually includes the:
   A. patient's name and identification number
   B. physician's name
   C. patient's bed assignment
   D. all of the above

 KNOWLEDGE LEVEL = 1

3. If an inpatient does not have an identification bracelet, who should be asked to make the identification before a venipuncture?
   A. a family member
   B. the patient
   C. the clerk who checked the patient in
   D. the nurse in charge of the patient

 KNOWLEDGE LEVEL = 1

4. A requisition for laboratory tests, whether computerized or handwritten, should contain the:
   A. patient's full name, identification number, and date of birth
   B. dates and types of tests to be performed
   C. physician's name
   D. all of the above

 KNOWLEDGE LEVEL = 1

5. The preferred position for a hospitalized patient during a venipuncture procedure is:
   A. sitting
   B. reclining
   C. standing
   D. none of the above

 KNOWLEDGE LEVEL = 1

6. Identify the most common site(s) for venipuncture.
   A. median cubital vein
   B. cephalic vein
   C. basilic vein
   D. all of the above

 KNOWLEDGE LEVEL = 1

7. Select one reason for not using arm veins for a venipuncture.
   A. The patient has IV lines or casts on both arms.
   B. The patient is a child.
   C. The patient is elderly.
   D. none of the above

 KNOWLEDGE LEVEL = 1

8. If arm veins cannot be used for a venipuncture, the preferred alternative veins lie in the:
   A. ankles or feet
   B. anterior surface of the hand or wrist

C. dorsal side of the hand or wrist

D. none of the above

 KNOWLEDGE LEVEL = 1

9. Which of the following must be included on the label of the blood specimen or body fluid specimen?

A. patient's name and identification number

B. the time that specimen is collected

C. the attending physician's name

D. all of the above

 KNOWLEDGE LEVEL = 1

10. If the tourniquet pressure is too tight or prolonged on the arm, what laboratory test result will be falsely elevated?

A. cell counts

B. protein

C. potassium

D. all of the above

 KNOWLEDGE LEVEL = 1

11. Where should the tourniquet be placed on the patient during the venipuncture procedure?

A. 1 inch above the venipuncture site

B. over the venipuncture site

C. 3 inches above the venipuncture site

D. 3 inches below the venipuncture site

 KNOWLEDGE LEVEL = 1

12. The most important information on the patient's identification bracelet that can be used as sole confirmation for identification purposes is the:

A. patient's name

B. hospital identification number

C. room number, bed assignment, and physician's name

D. address and telephone number

 KNOWLEDGE LEVEL = 1

13. Which of the following methods involves the use of a barrel and plunger to create a vacuum during venipuncture?

A. syringe method

B. tourniquet

C. capillary tube

D. evacuated tube method

 KNOWLEDGE LEVEL = 1

14. Which of the following causes pooling of blood in veins?

A. syringe method

B. tourniquet

C. capillary tube

D. evacuated tube method

 KNOWLEDGE LEVEL = 1

15. Which of the following methods requires a double-pointed needle?

A. syringe method

B. tourniquet

C. capillary tube

D. evacuated tube method

 KNOWLEDGE LEVEL = 1

16. During a venipuncture procedure, a tourniquet should not be left on a patient more than:

A. 10 seconds

B. 1 minute

C. 3 minutes

D. 4 minutes

KNOWLEDGE LEVEL = 1

17. Alcohol should be allowed to dry for how many seconds before the venipuncture?
    A. up to 5 seconds
    B. 6 to 10 seconds
    C. 10 to 15 seconds
    D. 30 to 60 seconds

 KNOWLEDGE LEVEL = 1

18. During the venipuncture, the needle should be inserted at what angle to the skin?
    A. 5 degree
    B. 15 degree
    C. 45 degree
    D. 90 degree

 KNOWLEDGE LEVEL = 1

19. During the venipuncture procedure, after the needle is inserted and blood begins to flow, what should the phlebotomist do next?
    A. Release the tourniquet.
    B. Withdraw the needle.
    C. Release the adapter.
    D. Adjust the hub of the needle.

 KNOWLEDGE LEVEL = 1

20. When the evacuated tube method is used for venipuncture, select the correct order of collection for the following tubes: blood culture tubes, coagulation tube, and hematology tube. Choose the order of tubes by their color of stoppers.
    A. light blue, lavender, yellow blood culture tubes
    B. lavender, light blue, yellow blood culture tubes

C. yellow blood culture tubes, blue, lavender
D. light blue, yellow blood culture tubes, lavender

 KNOWLEDGE LEVEL = 1

21. Which of the following information is essential for labeling a patient's specimen?
    A. the patient's name and identification number, date of collection, room number, and phlebotomist's initials
    B. the patient's name and identification number, date of collection, time of collection
    C. the patient's name and identification number, date and time of collection, phlebotomist's initials
    D. the patient's name and identification number, date of collection, physician's name

 KNOWLEDGE LEVEL = 1

22. The term "STAT" refers to:
    A. abstaining from food over a period of time
    B. using timed blood collections for specific specimens
    C. using the early morning specimens for laboratory testing
    D. immediate and urgent specimen collection

 KNOWLEDGE LEVEL = 1

23. Decontamination of a venipuncture site and the phlebotomist's gloved finger:
    A. increases blood flow to the skin
    B. removes dirt and prevents microbial contamination of the patient and specimen
    C. causes irritation to the patient's skin
    D. all of the above

KNOWLEDGE LEVEL = 1

24. Povidone-iodine (Betadine) preparations are used for:
    A. reducing the pain of the needle stick
    B. decontamination of the venipuncture site for all routine venipunctures
    C. decontamination of the venipuncture site for blood culture specimens
    D. all of the above

 KNOWLEDGE LEVEL = 1

25. Which of the following patients' emotional factors can have a negative effect on the blood collection process?
    A. nervousness or anxiety
    B. humor
    C. failure to wash hands
    D. none of the above

 KNOWLEDGE LEVEL = 1

26. Why is it important to get information about whether or not the patient has recently eaten?
    A. Laboratory tests can be affected by the ingestion of food and drink.
    B. Meals tend to calm a patient down.
    C. After eating, patients usually have enlarged veins.
    D. It is not important to get this information.

 KNOWLEDGE LEVEL = 1

27. How often should a health care worker's hands be washed when duties require that many patients' venipunctures be performed during a short period of time?
    A. after every two patients
    B. after every five patients
    C. at the beginning and end of a shift
    D. before and after each patient

 KNOWLEDGE LEVEL = 1

28. Steps in the hand-washing process should include:
    A. lathering with soap and water
    B. washing between the fingers and on the wrist area
    C. use of a foot pedal or clean paper towel to turn off the water faucet
    D. all of the above

 KNOWLEDGE LEVEL = 1

29. If a patient is obese, what special equipment, if any, would be helpful in the specimen collection process?
    A. specially sized collection tubes
    B. an oxygen mask
    C. a large-sized blood pressure cuff
    D. none of the above

 KNOWLEDGE LEVEL = 1

30. If a hospitalized patient is severely burned and cannot tolerate a hospital armband, what alternatives do phlebotomists have in confirming positive identification of the patient?
    A. Use the identification attached to the bed.
    B. Consult with any nurse on the unit.
    C. Check the room number and bed assignment.
    D. all of the above

KNOWLEDGE LEVEL = 2

31. After a health care worker has identified the patient and is setting up the supplies for a venipuncture procedure, what other types of information are important and helpful to the process?
    A. explanation of the reason for the encounter
    B. indication that it might be painful
    C. ascertaining whether or not the patient has eaten or drunk
    D. all of the above

 KNOWLEDGE LEVEL = 2

32. When a patient has "difficult" veins, what strategies, if any, can be used to improve the likelihood of a successful puncture?
    A. slight rotation of the patient's arm to a different position
    B. palpating the entire anticubital area to trace vein path
    C. warming the site
    D. all of the above

 KNOWLEDGE LEVEL = 2

33. Why is one side of the wrist more suitable for venipuncture than the other?
    A. Nerves lie close to the palmar side and can easily be injured.
    B. Veins are larger on the back side of the hand.
    C. On the palmer side, one can more easily feel an artery.
    D. all of the above

 KNOWLEDGE LEVEL = 2

34. Arteries differ from veins in which of the following ways?
    A. thicker vessel walls with a pulsating feel
    B. more blue in color
    C. smaller in diameter
    D. none of the above

 KNOWLEDGE LEVEL = 1

35. Acceptable alternatives to using a soft rubber tourniquet for the venipuncture procedure would include:
    A. string or cord
    B. blood pressure cuff
    C. rubber band
    D. all of the above

 KNOWLEDGE LEVEL = 1

36. During a venipuncture procedure, the needle should always be inserted with the:
    A. bevel side down
    B. bevel side up
    C. bevel pointed away from the insertion site
    D. none of the above

 KNOWLEDGE LEVEL = 2

37. When is a syringe method preferred over the evacuated tube method?
    A. when the patient has "difficult" veins
    B. when the family requests it
    C. when the patient has an IV in one arm
    D. all of the above

KNOWLEDGE LEVEL = 2

38. The winged infusion set is useful in venipunctures when:
   A. patients have small hand or wrist veins
   B. patients are young children
   C. patients are severely burned
   D. all of the above

 KNOWLEDGE LEVEL = 2

39. As one is withdrawing a needle from a patient's arm, what step should be considered *immediately*?
   A. activating the safety device on the needle
   B. applying an adhesive bandage to the site
   C. labeling the specimen
   D. disposing of the needle

 KNOWLEDGE LEVEL = 2

40. On occasion, specimens need to be rejected from laboratory testing. Which of the following factors may be used in this decision?
   A. The specimen is improperly transported.
   B. The specimen appears hemolyzed.
   C. The anticoagulated specimen contains blood clots.
   D. all of the above

 KNOWLEDGE LEVEL = 2

41. In drawing blood for multiple laboratory tests, why is it recommended that at least one other tube be drawn before the tubes for coagulation tests?
   A. to make sure that the coag tube is properly filled
   B. to reduce the chances of contaminating the specimen with tissue fluids
   C. to draw in the order that the tests will be performed in the laboratory
   D. to ensure that the needle does not fall out

 KNOWLEDGE LEVEL = 2

42. When collecting blood in a syringe, blood should be placed in the specimen tubes in the correct order to minimize contamination or clotting. The recommended order is:
   A. coagulation tubes, anticoagulated tubes, then blood culture tubes
   B. blood culture tubes, coagulation tubes, other anticoagulated tubes, tubes without anticoagulant additives
   C. tubes without anticoagulants, blood cultures, coagulation tubes
   D. none of the above

 KNOWLEDGE LEVEL = 1

43. List causes of hemolysis, if any, in a blood specimen drawn in a syringe.
   A. forcefully expelling blood into a tube from the syringe
   B. leaving the tourniquet on too long
   C. exposure to bright light
   D. none of the above

 KNOWLEDGE LEVEL = 1

44. The most commonly requested timed specimen is:
   A. glucose level
   B. cholesterol level
   C. triglycerides
   D. none of the above

 KNOWLEDGE LEVEL = 1

45. Peak and trough levels are useful for what type of analyses?
   A. hormone levels
   B. therapeutic drug levels
   C. glucose screening
   D. all of the above

KNOWLEDGE LEVEL = 1

46. The term "butterfly" refers to the:
    A. safety device on a needle
    B. evacuated collection tube
    C. winged infusion set
    D. all of the above

 KNOWLEDGE LEVEL = 1

47. All specimens should be handled:
    A. as if the specimens are sterile
    B. as if the specimens are hazardous and infectious
    C. as if the specimens are chemically clean
    D. all of the above

 KNOWLEDGE LEVEL = 2

Use the following scenario to refer to when answering Questions 48–50:

A health care worker entered a patient's room to draw blood specimens for the following tests: hematology cell counts, coagulation tests, blood cultures, and chemistry assays. The patient was an oncology patient and had scarring on many of her veins, had IVs in both forearms, and was a diabetic. Laboratory notes indicated that blood should not be drawn from this patient's feet. Answer the following questions about this scenario, assuming that an evacuated tube method would be used.

 KNOWLEDGE LEVEL = 2

48. Which site would be most suitable for blood collection?
    A. earlobe
    B. heel of the foot
    C. posterior side of the hand or wrist
    D. none of the above

 KNOWLEDGE LEVEL = 2

49. What would be the preferred order of tube collection for these tests?
    A. blood cultures, coagulation, hematology, and chemistry
    B. blood cultures, chemistry, hematology, and coagulation
    C. hematology, coagulation, chemistry, and blood cultures
    D. coagulation, blood cultures, hematology, and coagulation

 KNOWLEDGE LEVEL = 2

50. What measures could be taken to diminish the likelihood of complications?
    A. Use a butterfly system.
    B. Select the site carefully.
    C. Document the condition of the patient.
    D. all of the above

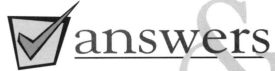

answers & rationales

1.

A. A hospitalized patient must be correctly identified by using his or her identification bracelet. A two-step identification process would involve the health care worker asking the patient his or her name, then confirming by checking the armband. (p. 232)

B. Positive identification of a hospitalized patient cannot be made by using the hospital room number and bed assignment because they are often the last to be changed when patients are discharged or new patients are admitted.

C. Identification using confirmation from a patient's relative for a hospitalized patient may be acceptable if it is confirmed by a nurse or by the identification armband.

D. "None of the above" is an incorrect answer.

2.

A. In addition to the patient's first and last names and identification number, the hospital identification bracelet may also include the patient's room number, bed assignment, and physician's name.

B. In addition to the patient's first and last names and identification number, the hospital identification bracelet may also include the patient's room number, bed assignment, and physician's name.

C. In addition to the patient's first and last names and identification number, the hospital identification bracelet may also include the patient's room number, bed assignment, and physician's name.

D. In addition to the patient's first and last names and identification number, the hospital identification bracelet may also include the patient's room number, bed assignment, and physician's name. (p. 232)

3.

A. A family member may identify the patient; however, the identity must be confirmed by a nurse in charge before a phlebotomy procedure is performed.

B. The patient may identify himself or herself; however, the identity must be confirmed by a nurse in charge before a phlebotomy procedure is performed.

C. Clerical personnel are not usually responsible for making positive identifications for hospitalized patients unless confirmed by a nurse in charge.

D. If a hospitalized patient does not have an identification bracelet, the nurse in charge of the patient should be asked to make the positive identification. This should be well documented. (p. 234)

4.

A. Laboratory requisitions for clinical testing, whether computerized or handwritten, must contain the patient's full name, identification number, and date of birth; the dates and types of tests to be performed; the physician's name, the location of the patient, and timing instructions.

B. Laboratory requisitions for clinical testing, whether computerized or handwritten, must contain the patient's full name, identification number, and date of birth; the dates and types of tests to be performed; the physician's name, the location of the patient, and timing instructions.

C. Laboratory requisitions for clinical testing, whether computerized or handwritten, must contain the patient's full name, identification number, and date of birth; the dates and types of tests to be performed; the physician's name, the location of the patient, and timing instructions.

D. Laboratory requisitions for clinical testing, whether computerized or handwritten, must contain the patient's full name, identification number, and date of birth; the dates and types of tests to be performed; the physician's name, the location of the patient, and timing instructions. (p. 234)

5.

A. A sitting position may be acceptable if the patient is in a comfortable chair with arm supports; however, it is important to remember that many hospitalized patients are weak and frail.

B. A reclining (supine) position for a hospitalized patient is generally preferred for phlebotomy because a patient who feels weak or faint will not fall or injure himself or herself while reclining. (p. 238)

C. A standing position for the patient is not acceptable for the performance of a phlebotomy procedure.

D. "None of the above" is an incorrect answer.

6.

A. The most common sites for venipuncture are in the antecubital area of the arm, where the median cubital vein, the cephalic vein, and the basilic vein lie close to the surface of the skin and are often prominent.

B. The most common sites for venipuncture are in the antecubital area of the arm, where the median cubital vein, the cephalic vein, and the basilic vein lie close to the surface of the skin and are often prominent.

C. The most common sites for venipuncture are in the antecubital area of the arm, where the median cubital vein, the cephalic vein, and the basilic vein lie close to the surface of the skin and are often prominent.

D. The most common sites for venipuncture are in the antecubital area of the arm, where the median cubital vein, the cephalic vein, and the basilic vein lie close to the surface of the skin and are often prominent. (p. 238)

7.

A. If a patient has an intravenous (IV) line or casts on both arms, the arms should not be used for performing a venipuncture. If the IV line or cast is only on one arm, the other arm may be used for venipuncture. (p. 240)

B. If the patient is a child, a venipuncture can still be performed by using appropriate pediatric methodologies.

C. If the patient is elderly, a venipuncture can be performed by using appropriate communication strategies and accommodations for the situation.

D. "None of the above" is incorrect.

8.

A. Ankle or foot veins should only be used if arm veins and hand or wrist veins on the dorsal side are inaccessible. Most hospitals have special guidelines regarding phlebotomy procedures from the foot area because coagulation and vascular complications tend to be more troublesome in the lower extremities, especially for diabetic patients.

B. The anterior surface of the wrist has many nerves that can be damaged during venipuncture, and the procedure would be much more painful than other sites. It is not an acceptable site for venipuncture.

C. When arm veins cannot be used for venipuncture, the preferred site is the back of the hand or wrist, that is, the dorsal surface, *not* the palm side of the hand. (p. 240)

D. "None of the above" is incorrect.

9.

A. Specimens should be labeled immediately at the patient's bedside or ambulatory setting, and the labels should contain the patient's full name and identification number, the date and time of collection, and the health care worker's initials. Other information that is helpful but optional is the patient's room number, bed assignment, or outpatient status.

B. Specimens should be labeled immediately at the patient's bedside or ambulatory setting, and the labels should contain the patient's full name and identification number, the date and time of collection, and the health care worker's initials. Other information that is helpful but optional is the patient's room number, bed assignment, or outpatient status.

C. Specimens should be labeled immediately at the patient's bedside or ambulatory setting, and the labels should contain the patient's full name and identification number, the date and time of collection, and the health care worker's initials. Other information that is helpful but optional is the patient's room number, bed assignment, or outpatient status.

D. Specimens should be labeled immediately at the patient's bedside or ambulatory setting, and the labels should contain the patient's full name and identification number, the date and time of collection, and the health care worker's initials. Other information that is helpful but optional is the patient's room number, bed assignment, or outpatient status. (p. 254)

10.

A. If a tourniquet is left on for more than 1 minute, it becomes uncomfortable and may cause blood to become hemoconcentrated. This could affect numerous laboratory tests, causing results to be elevated. Among the tests that may be affected are cell counts, protein, and potassium levels.

B. If a tourniquet is left on for more than 1 minute, it becomes uncomfortable and may cause blood to become hemoconcentrated. This could affect numerous laboratory tests, causing results to be elevated. Among the tests that may be affected are cell counts, protein, and potassium levels.

C. If a tourniquet is left on for more than 1 minute, it becomes uncomfortable and may cause blood to become hemoconcentrated. This could affect numerous laboratory tests, causing results to be elevated. Among the tests that may be affected are cell counts, protein, and potassium levels.

D. If a tourniquet is left on for more than 1 minute, it becomes uncomfortable and may cause blood to become hemoconcentrated. This could affect numerous laboratory tests, causing results to be elevated. Among the tests that may be affected are cell counts, protein, and potassium levels. (p. 246)

11.

A. The tourniquet should not be just 1 inch over the venipuncture site because it might get in the way during the procedure.

B. The tourniquet should not be covering or over the venipuncture site.

C. A tourniquet should be applied about 3 inches above the venipuncture site. It should be tight but not painful and should be partially looped to allow for easy release with one hand. (p. 243)

D. The tourniquet should not be 3 inches below the venipuncture site because it would serve no useful purpose in that location.

12.

A. The patient's name is very important to confirm identification; however, there are instances in which individuals with the same name are being tested. Therefore it is important to rely on a unique identification number as well.

B. The most important information on the patient's identification bracelet that can be used as sole confirmation for identification purposes is the patient's unique hospital identification number. (p. 232)

C. Room number, bed assignment, and physician's name are useful items of information; however, they are not reliable sources of patient identification.

D. Address and telephone number are also useful items of information; however, they are not reliable sources of patient identification.

13.

A. Venipuncture using the syringe method is similar to other methods. Once the needle is in the vein, the syringe plunger can be drawn back slowly to create a vacuum until the required amount of blood is drawn. The syringe method uses graduated markings on the barrel to indicate the volume of blood withdrawn. (p. 250)

B. A tourniquet does not create a vacuum during venipuncture.

C. Capillary tubes do not create a vacuum and are not used during venipuncture.

D. The evacuated tube method for venipuncture does not use a barrel and plunger.

14.

A. The syringe method does not cause pooling of blood in the veins.

B. A tourniquet causes pooling or filling of blood in veins. Such pooling makes blood collection easier during a venipuncture procedure, regardless of the method used to withdraw blood from the vein. (p. 243)

C. A capillary tube does not cause pooling of blood in the veins.

D. The evacuated tube method does not cause pooling of blood in the veins.

15.

A. The syringe method does not require a double-pointed needle.

B. Tourniquets do not require a double-pointed needle.

C. Capillary tubes do not require a double-pointed needle.

D. The evacuated tube method for venipuncture requires a double-pointed needle. The outside needle punctures the patient's vein, and the inside needle punctures the stopper of the collection tube. (pp. 247, 250)

16.

A. Ten seconds is not long enough to allow the blood to fill the vein.

B. A tourniquet should not be left on the patient's arm for more than 1 minute. It may be released and then reapplied, however; again the time should not exceed 1 minute. (p. 246)

C. Three minutes is too long to leave the tourniquet on because it is painful and uncomfortable and causes hemoconcentration.

D. Four minutes is too long to leave the tourniquet on because it is painful and uncomfortable and causes hemoconcentration.

17.

A. The alcohol will not dry in 5 seconds or less.

B. The alcohol will not dry in 6 to 10 seconds.

C. The alcohol will not dry in 10 to 15 seconds.

D. Alcohol should be allowed to dry for 30 to 60 seconds or should be wiped off with sterile gauze or cotton after the site is prepared. If the site is not dry, the alcohol will cause it to sting and/or may interfere with test results such as blood alcohol levels. (p. 247)

18.

A. A 5 degree angle is not adequate to reach the vein and penetrate the skin properly.

B. The needle should be inserted in the same direction as the vein at a 15 degree angle to the skin. (p. 247)

C. A 45 degree angle might cause the needle to go too deeply into the arm.

D. A 90 degree angle might cause the needle to go too deeply into the arm also.

19.

A. After the needle is inserted and blood begins to flow, the tourniquet should be released, and the patient may open his or her fist. (p. 247)

B. The needle should not be withdrawn until all blood specimens have been collected in the appropriate tubes.

C. Releasing the adaptor is not an appropriate action.

D. Adjusting the hub of the needle is not usually necessary unless it was not properly attached before venipuncture.

20.

A. Blood culture tubes should always be drawn first, in this case followed by coagulation tubes and then hematology tubes.

B. See A.

C. Blood culture tubes (yellow stoppers) are always collected first to reduce the chances of contamination. The coagulation tube (light blue stopper) should then be collected before the hematology tube (lavender stopper). (p. 253)

D. See A.

21.

A. The patient's room number, bed assignment, physician, or outpatient status is optional but useful information.

B. This information is incomplete; it is missing the phlebotomist's initials.

C. All specimen labels should include the patient's name and identification number, the date and time of collection, and the phlebotomist's initials. The patient's room number, bed assignment, or outpatient status is optional but useful information. (p. 254)

D. This information is incomplete; it is missing the time of collection and the phlebotomist's initials. The physician's name is useful but not required on a specimen label.

22.

A. Abstaining from food over a period of time is fasting.

B. Using timed blood collections is important for certain types of laboratory tests but does not refer to the term "STAT."

C. Using early morning specimens is typical for most hospital laboratories and is usually the routine procedure, not a "STAT" situation.

D. The term "STAT" refers to an immediate or emergency condition. It indicates that a patient has a medical condition that is critical or likely to become critical. STAT blood collections should be drawn and analyzed immediately. (p. 260)

23.

A. Decontamination does not increase blood flow to the skin.

B. Decontaminating the venipuncture site with a sterile swab or sponge containing 70 percent isopropanol removes dirt and prevents microbiological contamination of the patient and specimen. (p. 246)

C. Decontamination does not usually cause irritation to the patient's skin. Some patients are allergic to povidone-iodine, in which case other methods of decontamination can be used.

D. "All of the above" is not a correct answer.

24.

A. Iodine does not reduce the pain of the needlestick.

B. Iodine may be used for the decontamination step of a venipuncture site for any routine venipunctures; however, more patients are allergic to it than to isopropanol, it takes more time to use, and it is not cost effective.

C. Povidone-iodine preparations are used primarily for decontaminating the skin before venipuncture for blood gas analysis and blood cultures. Excess iodine should be removed from the skin with sterile gauze before the puncture. (p. 247)

D. "All of the above" is incorrect.

25.

A. Excessively anxious or emotional patients may need extra time to calm down before, during, or after the procedure. The phlebotomist should be aware of these emotional needs and know how to deal with them appropriately. (p. 231)

B. Humor is often helpful to the venipuncture process by relieving anxiety.

C. Failure to wash hands on the part of the phlebotomist is detrimental but is not an emotional factor or responsibility of the patient.

D. "None of the above" is incorrect.

26.

A. Many laboratory tests can be affected by the ingestion of food and drink. It is important to note whether or not the patient has been fasting. (p. 231)

B. Meals are usually enjoyable but do not necessarily calm a patient down, especially before a venipuncture.

C. Eating does not cause patients to have enlarged veins.

D. It is very important to get this information.

27.

A. Hand washing only after every two patients could result in transmission of infections and is not an acceptable practice.

B. Hand washing only after every five patients could result in transmission of infections and is not an acceptable practice.

C. Hand washing only at the beginning and end of a shift could result in transmission of infections and is not an acceptable practice.

D. Hands should be washed before and after each patient's specimen collection procedure. (p. 229)

28.

A. Hand-washing techniques should include lathering using soap and water; friction between hands, fingers, and wrist areas; and thorough rinsing until all soap is removed. The use of a foot pedal or clean paper towel to turn off the water faucet is also recommended.

B. Hand-washing techniques should include lathering using soap and water; friction between hands, fingers, and wrist areas; and thorough rinsing until all soap is removed. The use of a foot pedal or clean paper towel to turn off the water faucet is also recommended.

C. Hand-washing techniques should include lathering using soap and water; friction between hands, fingers, and wrist areas; and thorough rinsing until all soap is removed. The use of a foot pedal or clean paper towel to turn off the water faucet is also recommended.

D. Hand-washing techniques should include lathering using soap and water; friction between hands, fingers, and wrist areas; and thorough rinsing until all soap is removed. The use of a foot pedal or clean paper towel to turn off the water faucet is also recommended. (pp. 230–231)

29.

A. Collection tubes should be the same ones used for other routine testing.

B. An oxygen mask would not facilitate the venipuncture procedure.

C. Obese patients may require special equipment to facilitate the venipuncture procedure. This might include a large-sized blood pressure cuff to be used as a tourniquet and/or a longer needle for deeper penetration through the fatty layers to the vein. (p. 232)

D. "None of the above" is incorrect.

30.

A. In rare cases in which a patient is severely burned and cannot tolerate an identification armband, the phlebotomist may use the identification attached to the bed to make the confirmation. This step should be followed by a confirmation from the nurse in charge of that patient. (p. 234)

B. Consulting with any nurse on the unit may not be acceptable. It should be the nurse in charge of the patient.

C. Checking the room number and bed assignment is not an acceptable method of confirming identification because these are often changed when patients are admitted or discharged.

D. "All of the above" is incorrect.

31.

A. After introducing himself or herself, the health care worker may need to provide an explanation of the reason for the encounter or the types of tests the physician ordered. The procedure may need to be explained, including the fact that it might be painful. It is also important to ascertain whether or not the patient has eaten or drunk anything.

B. After introducing himself or herself, the health care worker may need to provide an explanation of the reason for the encounter or the types of tests the physician ordered. The procedure may need to be explained, including the fact that it might be painful. It is also important to ascertain whether or not the patient has eaten or drunk anything.

C. After introducing himself or herself, the health care worker may need to provide an explanation of the reason for the encounter or the types of tests the physician ordered. The procedure may need to be explained, including the fact that it might be painful. It is also important to ascertain whether or not the patient has eaten or drunk anything.

D. After introducing himself or herself, the health care worker may need to provide an explanation of the reason for the encounter or the types of tests the physician ordered. The procedure may need to be explained, including the fact that it might be painful. It is also important to ascertain whether or not the patient has eaten or drunk anything. (p. 237)

32.

A. To increase the likelihood of a successful puncture, several tips may help. These include slight rotation of the patient's arm to a different position, palpating the entire anticubital area to trace vein path, warming the site, gentle massaging, lowering the arm over the bedside, or using the other arm.

B. To increase the likelihood of a successful puncture, several tips may help. These include slight rotation of the patient's arm to a different position, palpating the entire anticubital area to trace vein path, warming the site, gentle massaging, lowering the arm over the bedside, or using the other arm.

C. To increase the likelihood of a successful puncture, several tips may help. These include slight rotation of the patient's arm to a different position, palpating the entire anticubital area to trace vein path, warming the site, gentle massaging, lowering the arm over the bedside, or using the other arm.

D. To increase the likelihood of a successful puncture, several tips may help. These include slight rotation of the patient's arm to a different position, palpating the entire anticubital area to trace vein path, warming the site, gentle massaging, lowering the arm over the bedside, or using the other arm. (pp. 238, 248–249)

33.

A. For hand vein punctures, the posterior surface of the wrist is preferred because the veins are larger. It is not acceptable to puncture the anterior, or palmar, side. Nerves lie close to the palmar side and can easily be injured by needle probing. Also, on the palmer side, one can feel an artery pulsating.

B. For hand vein punctures, the posterior surface of the wrist is preferred because the veins are larger. It is not acceptable to puncture the anterior, or palmar, side. Nerves lie close to the palmar side and can easily be injured by needle probing. Also, on the palmer side, one can feel an artery pulsating.

C. For hand vein punctures, the posterior surface of the wrist is preferred because the veins are larger. It is not acceptable to puncture the anterior, or palmar, side. Nerves lie close to the palmar side and can easily be injured by needle probing. Also, on the palmer side, one can feel an artery pulsating.

D. For hand vein punctures, the posterior surface of the wrist is preferred because the veins are larger. It is not acceptable to puncture the anterior, or palmar, side. Nerves lie close to the palmar side and can easily be injured by needle probing. Also, on the palmer side, one can feel an artery pulsating. (p. 169)

34.

A. Arteries do not feel like veins. They have thicker vessel walls, pulsate, and are considered more elastic. (p. 242)

B. Veins are actually more blue in color.

C. Diameter of veins and arteries varies based on the location in the body.

D. "None of the above" is incorrect.

35.

A. A string or cord would likely cause discomfort.

B. A tourniquet or blood pressure cuff are acceptable for use in a venipuncture procedure. Many types are available on the market. (p. 243)

C. A rubber band would also likely cause discomfort because it might be too tight.

D. "All of the above" is incorrect.

36.

A. The needle should never be inserted with the bevel side down.

B. In a venipuncture procedure, the needle should always be inserted with the bevel side upward and directly above a prominent vein or slightly below the palpable vein. One can feel a slight "pop" as the needle enters the vein. (p. 247)

C. The needle should never be inserted with the bevel pointed away from the insertion site.

D. "None of the above" is incorrect.

37.

A. The syringe method is usually used when a patient has more difficult veins. It provides more control to the phlebotomist in withdrawing blood. This is particularly useful with fragile veins. (p. 249)

B. When the family requests a particular venipuncture method, most facilities will try to accommodate their requests; however, individual facilities may have policies about the use and availability of specific supplies and equipment.

C. The fact that the patient has an IV in one arm does not influence which method to use for venipuncture. Other factors must be considered in this scenario.

D. "All of the above" is incorrect.

38.

A. Winged infusion sets are used for particularly difficult venipunctures. This includes patients with small hand or wrist veins, patients who are young children, patients who are severely burned, geriatric patients, patients who have had numerous needle sticks (such as oncology patients), patients in restrictive positions (arthritis), and those with fragile skin and veins.

B. Winged infusion sets are used for particularly difficult venipunctures. This includes patients with small hand or wrist veins, patients who are young children, patients who are severely burned, geriatric patients, patients who have had numerous needle sticks (such as oncology patients), patients in restrictive positions (arthritis), and those with fragile skin and veins.

C. Winged infusion sets are used for particularly difficult venipunctures. This includes patients with small hand or wrist veins, patients who are young children, patients who are severely burned, geriatric patients, patients who have had numerous needle sticks (such as oncology patients), patients in restrictive positions (arthritis), and those with fragile skin and veins.

D. Winged infusion sets are used for particularly difficult venipunctures. This includes patients with small hand or wrist veins, patients who are young children, patients who are severely burned, geriatric patients, patients who have had numerous needle sticks (such as oncology patients), patients in restrictive positions (arthritis), and those with fragile skin and veins. (p. 251)

39.

A. Health care workers should be extra cautious as the needle is removed from the patient, and activating the safety device on the needle according to the manufacturer's instructions is the next step. There are varying methods of activating safety devices, so proper training and use are vital to keeping accidental needle sticks at a minimum. (p. 252)

B. Applying an adhesive bandage to the site is important toward the end of the encounter with the patient and after checking for bleeding. This is not the step immediately after needle withdrawal.

C. Labeling the specimen is also important toward the end of the encounter. This is not the step immediately after needle withdrawal.

D. Disposing of the needle and contaminated supplies is also important at the end of the encounter, but it is not the step immediately after needle withdrawal.

40.

A. Clinical laboratories usually establish guidelines for specimen rejection. In general the following factors are considered: improper transportation, hemolysis, anticoagulated specimens containing blood clots, inadequate volume in tube, unlabeled tubes, wrong collection tube, outdated supplies used, or visible contamination.

B. Clinical laboratories usually establish guidelines for specimen rejection, In general the following factors are considered: improper transportation, hemolysis, anticoagulated specimens containing blood clots, inadequate volume in tube, unlabeled tubes, wrong collection tube, outdated supplies used, or visible contamination.

C. Clinical laboratories usually establish guidelines for specimen rejection, In general the following factors are considered: improper transportation, hemolysis, anticoagulated specimens containing blood clots, inadequate volume in tube, unlabeled tubes, wrong collection tube, outdated supplies used, or visible contamination.

D. Clinical laboratories usually establish guidelines for specimen rejection, In general the following factors are considered: improper transportation, hemolysis, anticoagulated specimens containing blood clots, inadequate volume in tube, unlabeled tubes, wrong collection tube, outdated supplies used, or visible contamination. (pp. 258–259)

41.

A. The order of draw does not usually relate to proper filling.

B. Drawing the coagulation tubes after at least one other tube of blood diminishes the chances of contamination with tissue fluids, which may initiate the clotting sequence. However, recent studies suggest that accurate coagulation results may be obtained by using the first tube. Therefore the phlebotomist must use the procedure specified by the health care facility. (p. 253)

C. The order of draw does not dictate the order that the tests will be performed in the laboratory.

D. The order of draw does not influence the status of the needle.

42.

A. Blood culture tubes should always be drawn first.

B. The correct order of disposing blood into tubes after collecting blood in a syringe is blood culture tubes, coagulation tubes, other anticoagulated tubes, and tubes without anticoagulant additives. (p. 254)

C. Blood culture tubes should always be drawn first.

D. "None of the above" is incorrect.

43.

A. Forcefully expelling blood into a tube from the syringe can cause hemolysis. (p. 256)

B. Leaving the tourniquet on too long does not usually cause hemolysis but may cause erroneous results.

C. Exposure to bright light does not usually cause hemolysis when blood is drawn in a syringe.

D. "None of the above" is incorrect.

44.

A. The most commonly requested timed specimen is for glucose level determinations, and is drawn 2 hours after a meal. (p. 259)

B. Cholesterol levels are not usually timed tests; however, fasting information is needed.

C. Triglyceride tests are not usually timed tests; however, fasting information is helpful.

D. "None of the above" is incorrect.

45.

A. Hormone levels increase and decrease depending on the time of day, so it is important to note the time of specimen collection; however, they are not monitored by drawing peak and trough specimens.

B. Peak and trough levels of certain drugs are useful to monitor the therapeutic levels. (p. 259)

C. Peak and trough glucose levels are not usually ordered by physicians.

D. "All of the above" is incorrect.

46.

A. Safety devices on needles are not called butterflies.

B. An evacuated collection tube is not a butterfly.

C. A winged infusion set is often called a butterfly needle assembly. It is used for very small veins and/or particularly difficult veins. (p. 251)

D. "All of the above" is incorrect.

47.

A. Specimens should be handled carefully, since they may be infectious, not sterile.

B. All specimens should be handled as if they are hazardous and infectious. (p. 229)

C. Specimens should be handled carefully, since they may be infectious, not chemically clean.

D. "All of the above" is incorrect.

48.

A. The earlobe would not be a suitable site for venipuncture or specimen acquisition for the amount of blood needed.

B. The heel of the foot should not be used in this case because of the risk of infections of the lower extremities in diabetics.

C. The posterior side of the hand or wrist, below the site of the IV, could be used for venipuncture. The situation should be documented. (p. 240)

D. "None of the above" is incorrect.

49.

A. The preferred order of draw would be blood cultures, coagulation, hematology, and chemistry tubes. (p. 253)

B. This order is not preferred.

C. This order is not preferred.

D. This order is not preferred.

50.

A. All of the following measures could be used to diminish the likelihood of complications: use of a butterfly system, careful site selection, and documentation of the patient's condition to explain unusual results.

B. All of the following measures could be used to diminish the likelihood of complications: use of a butterfly system, careful site selection, and documentation of the patient's condition to explain unusual results.

C. All of the following measures could be used to diminish the likelihood of complications: use of a butterfly system, careful site selection, and documentation of the patient's condition to explain unusual results.

D. All of the following measures could be used to diminish the likelihood of complications: use of a butterfly system, careful site selection, and documentation of the patient's condition to explain unusual results. (p. 251)

9 Skin Puncture Procedures

chapter objectives

Upon completion of Chapter 9, the learner is responsible for the following:

➤ Describe reasons for performing a skin puncture procedure.

➤ Identify the proper sites for performing a skin puncture procedure.

➤ Explain why controlling the depth of the puncture is necessary.

➤ Describe the process of making a blood smear.

➤ Explain why blood from a skin puncture procedure is different from blood taken by venipuncture.

DIRECTIONS Each of the questions or incomplete statements below is followed by four suggested answers or completions. Select **one answer** that is best in each case.

 KNOWLEDGE LEVEL = 1

1. Alcohol that has not dried on a skin puncture can:
   A. prevent a round drop from forming
   B. cause hemolysis of blood cells
   C. cause erroneous results for some laboratory tests
   D. all of the above

 KNOWLEDGE LEVEL = 1

2. Steps that are identical for venipuncture and finger-stick procedures are:
   A. site selection
   B. greeting, identification, and hand washing
   C. withdrawing the specimen
   D. puncture technique

 KNOWLEDGE LEVEL = 1

3. Skin puncture techniques are most often used when:
   A. small amounts of blood are needed for testing
   B. the patient is anemic
   C. the patient is a neonate
   D. all of the above

 KNOWLEDGE LEVEL = 1

4. The finger-stick procedure involves which of the following steps?
   A. The patient's finger should be held firmly with the phlebotomist's thumb away from the puncture site.

   B. The puncture should be done in one sharp continuous movement.
   C. The puncture device should be perpendicular to the skin.
   D. all of the above

 KNOWLEDGE LEVEL = 1

5. Preferred skin puncture sites is/are:
   A. thumb
   B. second, third, and fourth fingers
   C. middle finger only
   D. pinky finger

 KNOWLEDGE LEVEL = 1

6. Refer to Figure 9.1 to answer this question. Which puncture is the preferred method for a finger stick?
   A. Part A of Figure 9.1.
   B. Part B of Figure 9.1.
   C. all of the above
   D. none of the above

 KNOWLEDGE LEVEL = 1

7. Before a skin puncture procedure, a health care worker should do which of the following?
   A. emotional preparation
   B. supply and equipment preparation
   C. hand washing and putting on clean gloves
   D. all of the above

FIGURE 9.1.

A.   B.

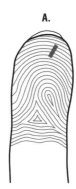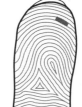

 KNOWLEDGE LEVEL = 1

8. Labeled skin puncture specimens should include the:
    A. patient's name and identification number
    B. time and date of collection
    C. phlebotomist's initials
    D. all of the above

 KNOWLEDGE LEVEL = 1

9. Which of the following conditions can have an adverse effect on the quality of a finger stick?
    A. the age of a patient
    B. the gender of a patient
    C. using the first drop of blood
    D. the presence of a wedding ring

 KNOWLEDGE LEVEL = 1

10. Blood smears for evaluation of cells must be made carefully. Which of the following features should not be present?
    A. one half of the slide being covered
    B. a feathered edge
    C. ridges and holes in the smear
    D. all of the above

 KNOWLEDGE LEVEL = 1

11. Skin puncture blood is composed of:
    A. tissue fluids
    B. blood from arterioles and venules
    C. blood from capillaries
    D. all of the above

 KNOWLEDGE LEVEL = 2

12. Skin puncture samples are often used for which of the following tests?
    A. white blood cell differentials
    B. blood cultures
    C. blood gases
    D. all of the above

 KNOWLEDGE LEVEL = 1

13. Which of the listed sequences is the best method for performing a finger stick?
    A. Squeeze the finger, decontaminate, puncture the skin.
    B. Decontaminate, squeeze the finger, puncture the skin, collect the first drop.
    C. Decontaminate, puncture the skin, wipe the first drop, collect the sample.
    D. Apply tourniquet, puncture the skin, wipe the first drop, collect the sample.

KNOWLEDGE LEVEL = 1

14. Warming a site for skin puncture:
    A. increases blood pressure
    B. increases blood flow to the site
    C. relaxes the patient
    D. eliminates the need for a tourniquet

 KNOWLEDGE LEVEL = 1

15. What should the phlebotomist do with the first drop of blood after a finger stick is performed?
    A. Use it for coagulation studies.
    B. Make a blood smear or slide.
    C. Wipe it off with gauze.
    D. Use it for hematology testing.

 KNOWLEDGE LEVEL = 1

16. What is the best angle for spreading a blood smear by using two glass slides?
    A. 15 degrees
    B. 30 degrees
    C. 45 degrees
    D. 90 degrees

 KNOWLEDGE LEVEL = 1

17. Which of the following should be used to decontaminate the site before skin puncture?
    A. isopropanol
    B. povidone-iodine
    C. diluted chlorox
    D. methanol

 KNOWLEDGE LEVEL = 1

18. What is the average depth a skin puncture should be for an adult?
    A. 0.5 to 1.0 mm
    B. 2 to 3 mm

C. 3 to 5 mm
D. 5.5 mm

 KNOWLEDGE LEVEL = 1

19. Excessive massaging or milking of the finger during a skin puncture procedure can cause:
    A. an adequate supply of blood for filling several capillary tubes
    B. increased venous blood flow to the puncture site
    C. hemolysis and contamination of the specimen with tissue fluids
    D. helpful results in glucose screening tests

 KNOWLEDGE LEVEL = 1

20. Osteomyelitis is defined as:
    A. infection of the blood
    B. infection of the spinal fluid
    C. inflammation and infection of the bone
    D. inflammation of the finger

 KNOWLEDGE LEVEL = 1

21. How does a capillary tube fill with blood during a skin puncture procedure?
    A. using suction from the collection device
    B. using the vacuum in the tube
    C. using capillary action
    D. using gravity

 KNOWLEDGE LEVEL = 1

22. In making a blood smear or slide, after the drop of blood has been spread across the glass slide, what is the next step?
    A. Gently blow on it to aid in drying.
    B. Hold it over a heating element to promote cellular adhesion to the glass.
    C. Add a drop of saline to the slide to preserve it.
    D. Allow it to air-dry.

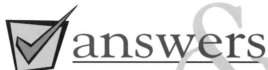

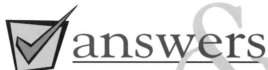answers & rationales

1.

A. The skin puncture site should be cleaned with 70 percent isopropanol and thoroughly dried before being punctured because residual alcohol causes rapid hemolysis and may contaminate glucose determinations. Alcohol also prevents round drops of blood from forming, which is needed for blood smear preparation.

B. The skin puncture site should be cleaned with 70 percent isopropanol and thoroughly dried before being punctured because residual alcohol causes rapid hemolysis and may contaminate glucose determinations. Alcohol also prevents round drops of blood from forming, which is needed for blood smear preparation.

C. The skin puncture site should be cleaned with 70 percent isopropanol and thoroughly dried before being punctured because residual alcohol causes rapid hemolysis and may contaminate glucose determinations. Alcohol also prevents round drops of blood from forming, which is needed for blood smear preparation.

D. The skin puncture site should be cleaned with 70 percent isopropanol and thoroughly dried before being punctured because residual alcohol causes rapid hemolysis and may contaminate glucose determinations. Alcohol also prevents round drops of blood from forming, which is needed for blood smear preparation. (p. 266)

2.

A. Site selection is different for the two procedures.

B. Steps that are identical for venipuncture and skin puncture procedures are greeting, identification, and hand washing. (pp. 264–265)

C. Withdrawing the specimen is different for the two procedures, especially in the types of supplies and physical maneuvers that are required by the phlebotomist.

D. The puncture technique is also different for the two procedures in that timing, feel/touch, and application of pressure vary significantly.

3.

A. Skin puncture techniques are most often used when small amounts of blood are needed for testing, when a patient is anemic, or complications may exist such as cardiac arrest, hemorrhage, venous thrombosis, reflex arteriospasm, gangrene of an extremity, danger to surrounding tissues or organs, infections, and injuries from restraining a child. Skin punctures are useful if the patient is a neonate, infant, or small child.

B. Skin puncture techniques are most often used when small amounts of blood are needed for testing, when a patient is anemic, or complications may exist such as cardiac arrest, hemorrhage, venous thrombosis, reflex arteriospasm, gangrene of an extremity, danger to surrounding tissues or organs, infections, and injuries from restraining a child. Skin punctures are useful if the patient is a neonate, infant, or small child.

C. Skin puncture techniques are most often used when small amounts of blood are needed for testing, when a patient is anemic, or complications may exist such as cardiac arrest, hemorrhage, venous thrombosis, reflex arteriospasm, gangrene of an extremity, danger to surrounding tissues or organs, infections, and injuries from restraining a child. Skin punctures are useful if the patient is a neonate, infant, or small child.

D. Skin puncture techniques are most often used when small amounts of blood are needed for testing, when a patient is anemic, or complications may exist such as cardiac arrest, hemorrhage, venous thrombosis, reflex arteriospasm, gangrene of an extremity, danger to surrounding tissues or organs, infections, and injuries from restraining a child. Skin punctures are useful if the patient is a neonate, infant, or small child. (p. 264)

4.

A. The finger-stick procedure involves holding a patient's finger firmly with the phlebotomist's thumb away from the puncture site. The puncture should be done in one sharp, continuous movement, and the puncture device should be held perpendicular to the skin (not at an angle) and punctured across the fingerprint.

B. The finger-stick procedure involves holding a patient's finger firmly with the phlebotomist's thumb away from the puncture site. The puncture should be done in one sharp, continuous movement, and the puncture device should be held perpendicular to the skin (not at an angle) and punctured across the fingerprint.

C. The finger-stick procedure involves holding a patient's finger firmly with the phlebotomist's thumb away from the puncture site. The puncture should be done in one sharp, continuous movement, and the puncture device should be held perpendicular to the skin (not at an angle) and punctured across the fingerprint.

D. The finger-stick procedure involves holding a patient's finger firmly with the phlebotomist's thumb away from the puncture site. The puncture should be done in one sharp, continuous movement, and the puncture device should be held perpendicular to the skin (not at an angle) and punctured across the fingerprint. (pp. 266–267)

5.

A. The thumb is not a preferred site for skin puncture. Positioning of the hand can be more awkward.

B. Preferred skin puncture sites are the fleshy portion of the second, third, and fourth fingers. (p. 265)

C. The middle finger is often used for skin puncture; however, it is not the only option.

D. The pinky finger is not recommended for skin puncture because the tissue of this finger is thinner than that of the others.

6.

A. Skin puncture is most effective if the puncture is made across the fingerprint. If the puncture is made along the lines of the fingerprint, the blood tends to run down the small grooves of the fingerprint and does not form a round drop of blood. (pp. 267–268)

B. This figure indicates a puncture made parallel to the fingerprint grooves. Blood from this puncture would not tend to form a nice round drop. More likely it would spread into the grooves and be more difficult to collect.

C. "All of the above" is incorrect.

D. "None of the above" is incorrect.

7.

A. Before performing a skin puncture, the health care worker should prepare himself or herself emotionally for the encounter, choose needed supplies and equipment, wash hands and put on clean gloves, and continue with the appropriate identification and greetings of the patient.

B. Before performing a skin puncture, the health care worker should prepare himself or herself emotionally for the encounter, choose needed supplies and equipment, wash hands and put on clean gloves, and continue with the appropriate identification and greetings of the patient.

C. Before performing a skin puncture, the health care worker should prepare himself or herself emotionally for the encounter, choose needed supplies and equipment, wash hands and put on clean gloves, and continue with the appropriate identification and greetings of the patient.

D. Before performing a skin puncture, the health care worker should prepare himself or herself emotionally for the encounter, choose needed supplies and equipment, wash hands and put on clean gloves, and continue with the appropriate identification and greetings of the patient. (pp. 264–265)

8.

A. Labeled skin puncture specimens should include the same information as on a venipuncture specimen, including the patient's name and identification number, the time and date of collection, and the phlebotomist's initials.

B. Labeled skin puncture specimens should include the same information as on a venipuncture specimen, including the patient's name and identification number, the time and date of collection, and the phlebotomist's initials.

C. Labeled skin puncture specimens should include the same information as on a venipuncture specimen, including the patient's name and identification number, the time and date of collection, and the phlebotomist's initials.

D. Labeled skin puncture specimens should include the same information as on a venipuncture specimen, including the patient's name and identification number, the time and date of collection, and the phlebotomist's initials. (p. 254)

9.

A. The age of a patient does not have an adverse effect on a skin puncture, even though the health care worker needs to consider special circumstances in dealing with elderly patients.

B. The gender of a patient does not have an adverse effect on a skin puncture.

C. Using the first drop of blood can have an adverse effect on a skin puncture specimen because it may be diluted with tissue fluids, thus causing erroneous results in laboratory tests. (pp. 268–269)

D. The presence of a wedding ring will not have an adverse effect on a skin puncture.

10.

A. Good blood smears should cover about one half of the slide.

B. Good blood smears have a feathered edge.

C. No ridges, lines, or holes should be present on a blood smear. (p. 269)

D. "All of the above" is incorrect.

11.

A. Skin puncture blood is composed of tissue fluids, blood from arterioles and venules, and blood from capillaries. The content of arterial blood is actually greater in skin puncture blood than of venous blood because the arterial pressure in the capillaries is stronger than the venous pressure.

B. Skin puncture blood is composed of tissue fluids, blood from arterioles and venules, and blood from capillaries. The content of arterial blood is actually greater in skin puncture blood than of venous blood because the arterial pressure in the capillaries is stronger than the venous pressure.

C. Skin puncture blood is composed of tissue fluids, blood from arterioles and venules, and blood from capillaries. The content of arterial blood is actually greater in skin puncture blood than of venous blood because the arterial pressure in the capillaries is stronger than the venous pressure.

D. Skin puncture blood is composed of tissue fluids, blood from arterioles and venules, and blood from capillaries. The content of arterial blood is actually greater in skin puncture blood than of venous blood because the arterial pressure in the capillaries is stronger than the venous pressure. (p. 264)

12.

A. Skin puncture samples are often used for white blood cell differentials. They are also used for a variety of screening tests (e.g., glucose, cholesterol) and other point-of-care procedures mentioned in Chapter 13. (p. 268)

B. Blood cultures are performed by venipuncture to minimize contamination and to acquire the amount of blood needed for detection of the infectious microorganisms.

C. Blood gases are usually evaluated using arterial samples.

D. "All of the above" is incorrect.

13.

A. The following steps are *not* in the correct order. Squeeze the finger, decontaminate, puncture the skin.

B. The following steps are *not* in the correct order: Decontaminate, squeeze the finger, puncture the skin, collect the first drop. Also, the first drop should be wiped off before collecting the sample.

C. The best method for performing a finger stick involves decontaminating the site, puncturing the skin, wiping the first drop, and collecting the sample. (pp. 264–265)

D. A tourniquet is not necessary in a skin puncture procedure.

14.

A. Warming a site for skin puncture does not increase blood pressure.

B. Warming a site for skin puncture increases blood flow to the site. (p. 265)

C. Warming a site for skin puncture does not necessarily relax the patient.

D. Warming a site for skin puncture has nothing to do with the need for a tourniquet, since tourniquets are not used for skin puncture procedures.

15.

A. The first drop of blood is not generally recommended for coagulation studies because it is mixed with tissue fluids.

B. The first drop of blood is not generally recommended for making a blood smear or slide because it is mixed with tissue fluids, so the blood is actually somewhat diluted.

C. After a finger stick is performed, the phlebotomist should wipe off the first drop of blood. (p. 266)

D. The first drop of blood is not generally recommended for hematology testing.

16.

A. 15 degrees is incorrect.

B. The best angle for spreading a blood smear using two glass slides is approximately 30 degrees. (p. 269)

C. 45 degrees is incorrect.

D. 90 degrees is incorrect.

17.

A. Isopropanol should be used to decontaminate the site before skin puncture. (p. 266)

B. Povidone-iodine may be used to decontaminate skin puncture sites under special circumstances; however, isopropanol is the recommended choice.

C. Diluted chlorox is not a recommended decontaminating agent for skin.

D. Methanol is not a recommended decontaminating agent for skin.

18.

A. A puncture depth of 0.5 to 1.0 mm may be too shallow to get adequate blood flowing for sample collection.

B. The average depth of a skin puncture should be 2 to 3 mm for an adult to avoid hitting the bone. (p. 268)

C. A puncture depth of 3 to 5 mm is too deep and may puncture the bone; this could lead to complications such as osteomyelitis.

D. A puncture depth of 5.5 mm is hazardous to the patient for the reasons mentioned above.

19.

A. Gentle massaging of the finger can assist in providing an adequate supply of blood for filling several capillary tubes; however, excessive massaging can damage the cells.

B. Excessive massaging or milking of the finger does not increase venous blood flow to the puncture site.

C. Excessive massaging or milking of the finger during a skin puncture procedure can cause hemolysis and contamination of the specimen with tissue fluids. (p. 268)

D. Excessive massaging or milking of the finger does not achieve helpful results in glucose screening tests; rather, it can cause erroneous results.

20.

A. Sepsis is an infection of the blood.

B. Meningitis is an infection of the spinal cord, fluid, and meninges.

C. Osteomyelitis is defined as inflammation and infection of the bone. (p. 268)

D. There is no specific term for inflammation of the finger.

21.

A. It is not necessary to use suction from the collection device when filling capillary tubes.

B. There is no vacuum in capillary tubes.

C. A capillary tube fills with blood during a skin puncture procedure using capillary action, whereby blood flows freely into the tube on contact without suction. (p. 268)

D. Capillary tubes do not require a downward position (for gravity to have an influence). However, blood flow from the finger may be better if the puncture site is held downward and gentle pressure is applied.

22.

A. Blood smears should never be blown on to aid in drying.

B. Blood smears should never be held over a heating element to promote cellular adhesion to the glass because cells may be destroyed in the process.

C. Blood smears do not require saline to preserve the cells.

D. In making a blood smear or slide, after the drop of blood has been spread across the glass slide, the next step is to allow it to air-dry and label it. (p. 269)

10 Complications in Blood Collection

chapter objectives

Upon completion of Chapter 10, the learner is responsible for the following:

➤ Describe physiologic and other complications related to phlebotomy procedures.

➤ Explain how to prevent complications in blood collection and how to handle the complications that do occur.

➤ List the effects of physical disposition on blood collection.

➤ Discuss the types of substances that can interfere in clinical analysis of blood constituents and the methods used to prevent these occurrences.

DIRECTIONS Each of the questions or incomplete statements below is followed by four suggested answers or completions. Select **one answer** that is best in each case.

 KNOWLEDGE LEVEL = 3

1. Which of the following analytes is significantly increased in the blood with changes in position?
   A. iron
   B. cortisol
   C. glucose
   D. testosterone

 KNOWLEDGE LEVEL = 1

2. A solid mass derived from blood constituents that occlude a blood vessel is/are:
   A. petechiae
   B. lymphostasis
   C. angiography
   D. thrombi

 KNOWLEDGE LEVEL = 2

3. If blood is to be collected for a timed blood glucose level determination, the patient must fast for:
   A. 4 to 6 hours
   B. 6 to 8 hours
   C. 8 to 12 hours
   D. 14 to 16 hours

 KNOWLEDGE LEVEL = 2

4. Which of the following laboratory test results are affected most if the patient is *not* fasting?
   A. cortisol
   B. testosterone
   C. triglycerides
   D. AST and CPK

 KNOWLEDGE LEVEL = 2

5. Emotional stress, such as anxiety or fear of blood collections, can lead to an increase in:
   A. serum iron
   B. blood glucose
   C. WBC count
   D. RBC count

 KNOWLEDGE LEVEL = 3

6. Upon entering Mrs. Hernandez's hospital room, the phlebotomist noticed that Mrs. Hernandez was taking three aspirin tablets. The patient commented that she was taking a second dose of aspirin because the first dose she took last night did not help her headache. What blood analyte will most likely be affected by the aspirin intake?
   A. glucose
   B. triglycerides
   C. ACTH
   D. bilirubin

 KNOWLEDGE LEVEL = 3

7. If the tourniquet is applied for longer than 3 minutes, which of the following analytes will most likely become falsely elevated?
   A. potassium
   B. bilirubin
   C. uric acid
   D. blood urea nitrogen

KNOWLEDGE LEVEL = 1

8. A basal state exists:
   A. before lunch
   B. after the evening meal
   C. in the early morning, 12 hours after the last ingestion of food
   D. in the afternoon, 3 hours after ingestion of lunch

 KNOWLEDGE LEVEL = 1

9. An abnormal accumulation of fluid in the intercellular spaces of the body that is localized or diffused is referred to as:
   A. hemoconcentration
   B. edema
   C. atherosclerosis
   D. hemolysis

 KNOWLEDGE LEVEL = 1

10. When the area around a venipuncture site starts to swell, this occurrence usually leads to:
    A. petechiae formation
    B. hematoma formation
    C. lymphostasis
    D. atherosclerosis

 KNOWLEDGE LEVEL = 3

11. Which of the following blood analytes is affected by diurnal rhythm?
    A. ACTH
    B. cholesterol
    C. creatinine
    D. CK

 KNOWLEDGE LEVEL = 1

12. When the phlebotomist collected blood from the patient, the patient was in a supine position. The patient was:
    A. standing
    B. lying
    C. sitting
    D. stooping

 KNOWLEDGE LEVEL = 3

13. The phlebotomist went to Patient Howell's hospital room to collect blood. The patient had already been transported to the cardiology unit for angiography. When the phlebotomist arrived at the cardiology unit, the patient had already undergone the angiography procedure. What blood laboratory test would be erroneously affected by the angiography procedure?
    A. cortisol
    B. RBC count
    C. WBC count
    D. reticulocyte count

 KNOWLEDGE LEVEL = 3

14. Which of the following blood analytes increases with age?
    A. estrogen
    B. cholesterol
    C. growth hormone
    D. glucose

 KNOWLEDGE LEVEL = 2

15. Another term for fainting is:
    A. fomite
    B. syncope
    C. lymphostasis
    D. thrombus

KNOWLEDGE LEVEL = 3

16. Falsely decreased laboratory test results for a blood analyte can be:
    A. mistakenly interpreted as normal when the blood analyte is truly in the subnormal range
    B. caused by increasing the color produced in the laboratory test
    C. mistakenly interpreted as normal or subnormal if the blood analyte is truly in an elevated range or normal range, respectively
    D. both A and B

 KNOWLEDGE LEVEL = 2

17. Which of the following should stop the health care worker from collecting blood from a patient's arm vein?
    A. heart attack that occurred the previous night
    B. cardiac bypass surgery
    C. high blood pressure
    D. mastectomy

 KNOWLEDGE LEVEL = 2

18. Which of the following has been shown to erroneously affect laboratory test results, leading to falsely elevated or decreased results?
    A. sneezing
    B. smiling
    C. violent crying
    D. syncope

 KNOWLEDGE LEVEL = 3

19. If a patient becomes extremely anxious and stressed during the blood collection procedure and begins to hyperventilate, which of the following laboratory results will become altered because of this stress?
    A. RBC count
    B. blood pH level
    C. triglyceride level
    D. protein level

 KNOWLEDGE LEVEL = 2

20. Which of the following would most likely *not* be an explanation for turbid serum?
    A. bacterial contamination
    B. elevated glucose results
    C. elevated cholesterol results
    D. elevated triglyceride results

 KNOWLEDGE LEVEL = 1

21. Figure 10.1 depicts:
    A. a woman's arm showing lymphostasis
    B. petechiae close to the antecubital
    C. a woman's arm showing hemoconcentration
    D. a hematoma appearing close to the antecubital fossa area

 KNOWLEDGE LEVEL = 2

22. Which of the following occurs as the result of inflammation and disease of the interstitial compartments?
    A. hemoconcentration
    B. sclerosed veins
    C. syncope
    D. hematoma

FIGURE 10.1.

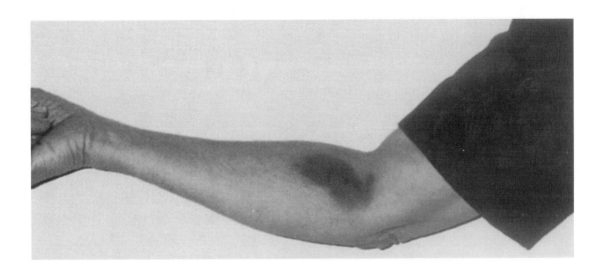

 KNOWLEDGE LEVEL = 3

23. Falsely increased laboratory results for a blood analyte can be:
    A. caused by a medication competing with the blood analyte for a chromogenic reagent, thus falsely decreasing the resultant color of the reaction
    B. mistakenly interpreted as elevated or normal if the blood analyte is truly in a normal range or a decreased range, respectively
    C. mistakenly interpreted as normal or subnormal if the blood analyte is truly in an elevated range or a normal range
    D. both A and C

 KNOWLEDGE LEVEL = 1

24. When hemoglobin is released and serum becomes tinged with pink or red, this condition is referred to as:
    A. hemoconcentration
    B. hemophilia
    C. hemolysis
    D. lymphocytosis

 KNOWLEDGE LEVEL = 3

25. If the phlebotomist notices that the patient is taking aspirin, the blood collector should ask whether the patient has informed his or her physician about taking aspirin, since aspirin can lead to erroneously decreased levels of blood analytes, including:
    A. ACTH
    B. bilirubin
    C. BUN
    D. total protein

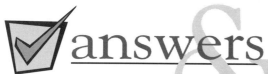

answers & rationales

1.

A. Changing from a lying position to a sitting or standing position causes body water to shift from intravascular to interstitial compartments (in tissues), and certain larger molecules such as iron cannot filter into the tissue. Thus they concentrate in the blood. (p. 282)

B. Changing from a lying position to a sitting or standing position causes body water to shift from intravascular to interstitial compartments (in tissues), and certain larger molecules such as iron cannot filter into the tissue. Thus they concentrate in the blood. However, cortisol is not significantly increased in the blood with changes in position.

C. Changing from a lying position to a sitting or standing position causes body water to shift from intravascular to interstitial compartments (in tissues), and certain larger molecules such as iron cannot filter into the tissue. Thus they concentrate in the blood. However, glucose is not significantly increased in the blood with changes in position.

D. Changing from a lying position to a sitting or standing position causes body water to shift from intravascular to interstitial compartments (in tissues), and certain larger molecules such as iron cannot filter into the tissue. Thus they concentrate in the blood. Testosterone is not significantly increased in the blood with changes in position.

2.

A. Petechiae are small red spots appearing on a patient's skin indicating that minute amounts of blood have escaped into skin epithelium.

B. Lymphostasis means no lymph flow and occurs because of lymph node removal adjacent to the breast.

C. Thrombi are solid masses derived from blood constituents that reside in the blood vessels.

D. Thrombi are solid masses derived from blood constituents that reside in the blood vessels. (p. 279)

3.

A. If blood is to be collected for a timed blood glucose level determination, the patient needs to fast for 8 to 12 hours. Prolonged fasting has been shown to falsely alter blood test results.

B. If blood is to be collected for a timed blood glucose level determination, the patient needs to fast for 8 to 12 hours. Prolonged fasting has been shown to falsely alter blood test results.

C. If blood is to be collected for a timed blood glucose level determination, the patient needs to fast for 8 to 12 hours. Prolonged fasting has been shown to falsely alter blood test results. (p. 280)

D. If blood is to be collected for a timed blood glucose level determination, the patient needs to fast for 8 to 12 hours. Prolonged fasting has been shown to falsely alter blood test results.

4.

A. Cortisol is a hormone, and the blood concentration is not affected by eating.

B. Testosterone is a hormone, and the blood concentration is not affected by eating.

C. If a patient has recently eaten fatty substances, he or she may have a temporarily elevated lipid level (i.e., triglycerides), and the serum will appear lipemic, or cloudy. (p. 281)

D. AST and CPK are enzymes and the blood concentrations are not affected by eating.

5.

A. Emotional stress, such as anxiety or fear of blood collection, can lead to a decrease in serum iron levels.

B. Blood glucose levels are not significantly altered because of emotional stress or anxiety.

C. Emotional stress, such as anxiety or fear of blood collection, can lead to an increase in the WBC count. (p. 281)

D. RBC counts are not significantly altered because of emotional stress or anxiety.

6.

A. Aspirin causes hypobiliruminemia (a decrease in bilirubin) by expelling bilirubin from the plasma to the surrounding tissue cells.

B. Aspirin causes hypobiliruminemia (a decrease in bilirubin) by expelling bilirubin from the plasma to the surrounding tissue cells.

C. Aspirin causes hypobiliruminemia (a decrease in bilirubin) by expelling bilirubin from the plasma to the surrounding tissue cells.

D. Aspirin causes hypobiliruminemia (a decrease in bilirubin) by expelling bilirubin from the plasma to the surrounding tissue cells. (p. 283)

7.

A. The pressure of the tourniquet causes potassium to leak from the tissue cells into the blood, leading to falsely elevated values if the tourniquet pressure is prolonged. (p. 282)

B. The pressure of the tourniquet causes potassium to leak from the tissue cells into the blood, leading to falsely elevated values if the tourniquet pressure is prolonged.

C. The pressure of the tourniquet causes potassium to leak from the tissue cells into the blood, leading to falsely elevated values if the tourniquet pressure is prolonged.

D. The pressure of the tourniquet causes potassium to leak from the tissue cells into the blood, leading to falsely elevated values if the tourniquet pressure is prolonged.

8.

A. Basal state exists in the early morning, approximately 12 hours after the last ingestion of food.

B. Basal state exists in the early morning, approximately 12 hours after the last ingestion of food.

C. Basal state exists in the early morning, approximately 12 hours after the last ingestion of food. (p. 280)

D. Basal state exists in the early morning, approximately 12 hours after the last ingestion of food.

9.

A. Hemoconcentration refers to an increased concentration of larger molecules and formed elements in the blood.

B. An abnormal accumulation of fluid in the intercellular spaces of the body that is localized or diffused is referred to as edema. (p. 278)

C. Atherosclerosis is the accumulation of fat deposits within the blood vessels.

D. Hemolysis is the breakdown of red blood cells, releasing hemoglobin into the plasma.

10.

A. Petechiae are small red spots appearing on a patient's skin and generally indicates that minute amounts of blood have escaped into skin epithelium.

B. When the area around the venipuncture site starts to swell, usually blood is leaking into the tissues and causing a hematoma. (p. 275)

C. Lymphostasis refers to no lymph flow.

D. Atherosclerosis is the accumulation of fat deposits within the blood vessels.

11.

A. Diurnal rhythms are body fluid fluctuations during the day that affect certain blood analytes such as ACTH. (p. 281)

B. Diurnal rhythms are body fluid fluctuations during the day that affect certain blood analytes such as ACTH.

C. Diurnal rhythms are body fluid fluctuations during the day that affect certain blood analytes such as ACTH.

D. Diurnal rhythms are body fluid fluctuations during the day that affect certain blood analytes such as ACTH.

12.

A. The patient was in the lying position.

B. The patient was in the lying position. (p. 281)

C. The patient was in the lying position.

D. The patient was in the lying position.

13.

A. Fluorescein angiography can erroneously alter the blood cortisol results. (p. 283)

B. Fluorescein angiography can erroneously alter the blood cortisol results.

C. Fluorescein angiography can erroneously alter the blood cortisol results.

D. Fluorescein angiography can erroneously alter the blood cortisol results.

14.

A. Estrogen levels decrease in geriatric women.

B. Blood cholesterol levels increase with age. (p. 282)

C. Growth hormone levels decrease with age.

D. Glucose levels are not affected by age.

15.

A. Another term for fainting is syncope.

B. Another term for fainting is syncope. (p. 224)

C. Lymphostasis refers to no lymph flow and occurs due to lymph node removal.

D. A thrombus is a solid mass derived from blood constituents that reside in blood vessels.

16.

A. Falsely decreased values of a blood analyte can be mistakenly interpreted as normal or subnormal if the blood analyte is truly in an elevated range or a normal range, respectively.

B. Falsely decreased values of a blood analyte can be mistakenly interpreted as normal or subnormal if the blood analyte is truly in an elevated range or a normal range, respectively.

C. Falsely decreased values of a blood analyte can be mistakenly interpreted as normal or subnormal if the blood analyte is truly in an elevated range or a normal range, respectively. (p. 283)

D. Falsely decreased values of a blood analyte can be mistakenly interpreted as normal or subnormal if the blood analyte is truly in an elevated range or a normal range, respectively.

17.

A. A woman or man who has had a mastectomy (removal of a breast) may also have lymphostasis due to lymph node removal adjacent to the breast. Without lymph flow on that particular side of the body, the patient is highly susceptible to infection, and some blood analytes may be altered. Therefore venipuncture should *not* be performed on the same side as that of a mastectomy.

B. A woman or man who has had a mastectomy (removal of a breast) may also have lymphostasis due to lymph node removal adjacent to the breast. Without lymph flow on that particular side of the body, the patient is highly susceptible to infection, and some blood analytes may be altered. Therefore venipuncture should *not* be performed on the same side as that of a mastectomy.

C. A woman or man who has had a mastectomy (removal of a breast) may also have lymphostasis due to lymph node removal adjacent to the breast. Without lymph flow on that particular side of the body, the patient is highly susceptible to infection, and some blood analytes may be altered. Therefore venipuncture should *not* be performed on the same side as that of a mastectomy.

D. A woman or man who has had a mastectomy (removal of a breast) may also have lymphostasis due to lymph node removal adjacent to the breast. Without lymph flow on that particular side of the body, the patient is highly susceptible to infection, and some blood analytes may be altered. Therefore venipuncture should *not* be performed on the same side as that of a mastectomy. (p. 277)

18.

A. Violent crying can falsely alter laboratory test results dramatically.

B. Violent crying can falsely alter laboratory test results dramatically.

C. Violent crying can falsely alter laboratory test results dramatically. (p. 281)

D. Violent crying can falsely alter laboratory test results dramatically.

19.

A. Anxiety that results in hyperventilation also causes acid-base imbalances, changing the blood pH level.

B. Anxiety that results in hyperventilation also causes acid-base imbalances, changing the blood pH level. (p. 281)

C. Anxiety that results in hyperventilation also causes acid-base imbalances, changing the blood pH level.

D. Anxiety that results in hyperventilation also causes acid-base imbalances, changing the blood pH level.

20.

A. Turbid serum appears cloudy or milky and can be a result of bacterial contamination or high lipid (i.e., cholesterol, triglyceride) levels in the blood.

B. Turbid serum appears cloudy or milky and can be a result of bacterial contamination or high lipid (i.e., cholesterol, triglyceride) levels in the blood. (p. 281)

C. Turbid serum appears cloudy or milky and can be a result of bacterial contamination or high lipid (i.e., cholesterol, triglyceride) levels in the blood.

D. Turbid serum appears cloudy or milky and can be a result of bacterial contamination or high lipid (i.e., cholesterol, triglyceride) levels in the blood.

21.

A. This woman's arm shows a hematoma close to the antecubital fossa area. A hematoma can occur when the needle has gone completely through a vein, the bevel opening is partially in the vein, or not enough pressure is applied to the site after puncture.

B. This woman's arm shows a hematoma close to the antecubital fossa area. A hematoma can occur when the needle has gone completely through a vein, the bevel opening is partially in the vein, or not enough pressure is applied to the site after puncture.

C. This woman's arm shows a hematoma close to the antecubital fossa area. A hematoma can occur when the needle has gone completely through a vein, the bevel opening is partially in the vein, or not enough pressure is applied to the site after puncture.

D. This woman's arm shows a hematoma close to the antecubital fossa area. A hematoma can occur when the needle has gone completely through a vein, the bevel opening is partially in the vein, or not enough pressure is applied to the site after puncture. (p. 275)

22.

A. Hemoconcentration is usually a complication of tourniquet application, massaging, squeezing, or probing a site.

B. Sclerosed, or hardened, veins are a result of inflammation and disease of the interstitial compartments. (p. 278)

C. Syncope is another term for fainting, which occurs occasionally in patients who are having blood collections.

D. Hematomas are the result of a needle puncture that has gone completely through the vein, the bevel opening is partially in the vein, or not enough pressure is applied to the site after puncture.

23.

A. Falsely increased laboratory test results for a blood analyte can be mistakenly interpreted as elevated or normal if the blood analyte is truly in a normal range or a decreased range, respectively.

B. Falsely increased laboratory test results for a blood analyte can be mistakenly interpreted as elevated or normal if the blood analyte is truly in a normal range or a decreased range, respectively. (p. 283)

C. Falsely increased laboratory test results for a blood analyte can be mistakenly interpreted as elevated or normal if the blood analyte is truly in a normal range or a decreased range, respectively.

D. Falsely increased laboratory test results for a blood analyte can be mistakenly interpreted as elevated or normal if the blood analyte is truly in a normal range or a decreased range, respectively.

24.

A. Hemoconcentration is an increased concentration of larger molecules and formed elements in the blood.

B. Hemophilia actually means "the love of red blood cells," which occurs in hemophiliacs, who lose large amounts of blood owing to clotting abnormalities.

C. Hemolysis is when the RBCs are lysed and release hemoglobin. (pp. 278–279)

D. Lymphocytosis refers to the white blood cells, lymphocytes, which do not contain hemoglobin. Hemoglobin is contained in erythrocytes, red blood cells.

25.

A. Aspirin causes hypobilirubinemia (a decrease in bilirubin) by expelling bilirubin from the plasma to the surrounding tissue cells.

B. Aspirin causes hypobilirubinemia (a decrease in bilirubin) by expelling bilirubin from the plasma to the surrounding tissue cells. (p. 283)

C. Aspirin causes hypobilirubinemia (a decrease in bilirubin) by expelling bilirubin from the plasma to the surrounding tissue cells.

D. Aspirin causes hypobilirubinemia (a decrease in bilirubin) by expelling bilirubin from the plasma to the surrounding tissue cells.

Special Procedures and Point-of-Care Testing

11 Pediatric Procedures

chapter objectives

Upon completion of Chapter 11, the learner is responsible for the following:

➤ Describe fears or concerns that children in different developmental stages might have toward the blood collection process.

➤ List suggestions that might be appropriate for parental behavior during a venipuncture or skin puncture.

➤ Identify puncture sites for a heel stick on an infant and demonstrate the procedure.

➤ Describe the venipuncture sites for infants and young children.

➤ Discuss the types of equipment and supplies that must be used during microcollection and venipuncture of infants and children.

➤ Describe the procedure for screening neonates for phenylketonuria (PKU).

DIRECTIONS Each of the questions or incomplete statements below is followed by four suggested answers or completions. Select **one answer** that is best in each case.

 KNOWLEDGE LEVEL = 1

1. EMLA is sometimes used for pediatric venipuncture procedures. EMLA is a:
   A. local anesthetic applied with a small needle to the child's arm before venipuncture
   B. topical anesthetic applied to the child's arm before venipuncture
   C. topical lotion applied to the child's arm after venipuncture to stop bleeding at the venipuncture site
   D. topical lotion applied to the child's arm before venipuncture to assist the phlebotomist in finding a vein

 KNOWLEDGE LEVEL = 2

2. The best location for performing a phlebotomy on a hospitalized child is:
   A. at the bedside in a chair
   B. in a playroom
   C. in a treatment room
   D. in his or her bed

 KNOWLEDGE LEVEL = 1

3. The optimal depth of a finger stick in a child is:
   A. greater than 3.0 mm
   B. less than 0.5 mm
   C. less than 0.24 mm
   D. less than 2.4 mm

 KNOWLEDGE LEVEL = 1

4. What needle gauge is required for scalp vein venipuncture of an infant?
   A. 17
   B. 19
   C. 21
   D. 23

 KNOWLEDGE LEVEL = 1

5. The angle of the needle for scalp vein venipuncture of an infant should be:
   A. 15 degrees
   B. 30 degrees
   C. 45 degrees
   D. 60 degrees

 KNOWLEDGE LEVEL = 2

6. Complications resulting from multiple deep skin punctures on an infant's heel include:
   A. hepatitis
   B. AIDS
   C. pneumonia
   D. osteomyelitis

 KNOWLEDGE LEVEL = 1

7. A commonly inherited disease that is detected through a blood screening process in neonates is:
   A. phenylketonuria
   B. spina bifida
   C. neurogenic bladder abnormality
   D. anemia

KNOWLEDGE LEVEL = 1

8. After a dorsal hand vein blood collection, pressure should be applied over the venipuncture site with a dry gauze sponge for:
   A. 20 to 30 seconds
   B. 30 to 60 seconds
   C. 1/2 to 1-1/2 minutes
   D. 2 to 3 minutes

 KNOWLEDGE LEVEL = 2

9. The dorsal hand vein technique for infants includes which of the following steps?
   A. The patient's wrist veins are used.
   B. The health care provider collecting the sample uses a small Velcro-type tourniquet.
   C. The infant is stuck with a safety lancet.
   D. Blood is collected directly from the hub of the needle.

 KNOWLEDGE LEVEL = 2

10. When a skin puncture is performed on an infant or a child, which of the following specimens is collected first?
    A. blood bank specimens
    B. chemistry specimens
    C. clinical immunology specimens
    D. hematology specimens

 KNOWLEDGE LEVEL = 2

11. A 10-mL blood sample taken from a premature or newborn infant is equivalent to what percent of the infant's total blood volume?
    A. 1 to 2 percent
    B. 3 to 4 percent
    C. 5 to 10 percent
    D. 10 to 15 percent

 KNOWLEDGE LEVEL = 1

12. Which of the following is needed for blood collection by skin puncture on an infant?
    A. puncture-resistant sharps container
    B. Safety-Lok needle holder
    C. purple-topped evacuated tube
    D. Velcro-type tourniquet

 KNOWLEDGE LEVEL = 2

13. The total blood volume of a premature infant is calculated by multiplying weight in kilograms by:
    A. 115 mL/kg
    B. 80–110 mL/kg
    C. 75–100 mL/kg
    D. 70 mL/kg

 KNOWLEDGE LEVEL = 1

14. Neonatal blood screening is required by law to test for:
    A. hypoadrenalism
    B. hypothyroidism
    C. spina bifida
    D. congenital neurogenic bladder anomaly

 KNOWLEDGE LEVEL = 1

15. After the blood is collected from the newborn for PKU testing, the card must dry in a horizontal position for a minimum of:
    A. 30 minutes
    B. 1 hour
    C. 2 hours
    D. 3 hours

KNOWLEDGE LEVEL = 2

16. When collecting blood from a saline lock on a child, the blood collector must check the patency of the line by:
    A. disinfecting the catheter cap with alcohol or povidone-iodine solution
    B. flushing with a small amount of normal saline
    C. injecting slowly the heparinized flush solution
    D. flushing with a small amount of glucose solution

 KNOWLEDGE LEVEL = 1

17. Which of the following is an acceptable intervention to alleviate pain during venipuncture on an infant or child?
    A. xylocaine
    B. sucrose nipple
    C. ice pack
    D. EMLA

 KNOWLEDGE LEVEL = 1

18. Which is the preferred site for a heel stick?
    A. anteromedial aspect
    B. medial or lateral aspect
    C. posterior curve
    D. a previous puncture site

 KNOWLEDGE LEVEL = 3

19. Which of the following is true concerning skin puncture on an infant compared with the dorsal hand venipuncture procedure?
    A. It is less stressful for the infant.
    B. There is less dilution of the specimen with tissue fluid.
    C. Hemolysis occurs more often.
    D. Fewer punctures are required.

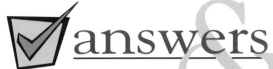

answers & rationales

1.

A. Eutectic mixture of local anesthetics (EMLA) is a topical anesthetic applied to the child's arm before venipuncture.

B. Eutectic mixture of local anesthetics (EMLA) is a topical anesthetic applied to the child's arm before venipuncture. (p. 303)

C. Eutectic mixture of local anesthetics (EMLA) is a topical anesthetic applied to the child's arm before venipuncture.

D. Eutectic mixture of local anesthetics (EMLA) is a topical anesthetic applied to the child's arm before venipuncture.

2.

A. For psychological reasons, the best room location for a painful procedure such as phlebotomy is a treatment room away from the child's bed or playroom.

B. For psychological reasons, the best room location for a painful procedure such as phlebotomy is a treatment room away from the child's bed or playroom.

C. For psychological reasons, the best room location for a painful procedure such as phlebotomy is a treatment room away from the child's bed or playroom. (p. 301)

D. For psychological reasons, the best room location for a painful procedure such as phlebotomy is a treatment room away from the child's bed or playroom.

3.

A. An automatic lancet should be used for the finger stick to a child, and the stick should not exceed 2.4 mm for small children.

B. An automatic lancet should be used for the finger stick to a child, and the stick should not exceed 2.4 mm for small children.

C. An automatic lancet should be used for the finger stick to a child, and the stick should not exceed 2.4 mm for small children.

D. An automatic lancet should be used for the finger stick to a child, and the stick should not exceed 2.4 mm for small children. (p. 311)

4.

A. A 23- or 25-gauge safety winged infusion set (butterfly needle) is used for the venipuncture.

B. A 23- or 25-gauge safety winged infusion set (butterfly needle) is used for the venipuncture.

C. A 23- or 25-gauge safety winged infusion set (butterfly needle) is used for the venipuncture.

D. A 23- or 25-gauge safety winged infusion set (butterfly needle) is used for the venipuncture. (p. 315)

5.

A. Position the needle at a 15 degree angle over the infant's scalp vein in the direction of the blood flow. (p. 316)

B. Position the needle at a 15 degree angle over the infant's scalp vein in the direction of the blood flow.

C. Position the needle at a 15 degree angle over the infant's scalp vein in the direction of the blood flow.

D. Position the needle at a 15 degree angle over the infant's scalp vein in the direction of the blood flow.

6.

A. Osteomyelitis can result from multiple deep skin punctures on an infant's heel.

B. Osteomyelitis can result from multiple deep skin punctures on an infant's heel.

C. Osteomyelitis can result from multiple deep skin punctures on an infant's heel.

D. Osteomyelitis can result from multiple deep skin punctures on an infant's heel. (p. 307)

7.

A. In the United States, neonatal blood screening for phenylketonuria (PKU) and hypothyroidism is mandatory by law. These diseases can result in severe abnormalities, including mental retardation. (p. 309)

B. Spina bifida is a congenital defect that is detected through a blood sample taken when the baby is still a fetus in the womb of the mother. Once the baby is born, the congenital abnormality is evident and not reversible.

C. In the United States, neonatal blood screening for phenylketonuria (PKU) and hypothyroidism is mandatory by law. These diseases can result in severe abnormalities, including mental retardation.

D. In the United States, neonatal blood screening for phenylketonuria (PKU) and hypothyroidism is mandatory by law. These diseases can result in severe abnormalities, including mental retardation.

8.

A. After the dorsal hand vein blood collection, pressure should be applied over the puncture site with a dry gauze sponge for 2 to 3 minutes.

B. After the dorsal hand vein blood collection, pressure should be applied over the puncture site with a dry gauze sponge for 2 to 3 minutes.

C. After the dorsal hand vein blood collection, pressure should be applied over the puncture site with a dry gauze sponge for 2 to 3 minutes.

D. After the dorsal hand vein blood collection, pressure should be applied over the puncture site with a dry gauze sponge for 2 to 3 minutes. (pp. 313–315)

9.

A. The dorsal hand vein technique for neonates and infants does not require the use of a tourniquet. The dorsal vein in the hand is used for the collection, and a needle is used to obtain the blood. The blood is collected directly from the hub of the needle.

B. The dorsal hand vein technique for neonates and infants does not require the use of a tourniquet. The dorsal vein in the hand is used for the collection, and a needle is used to obtain the blood. The blood is collected directly from the hub of the needle.

C. The dorsal hand vein technique for neonates and infants does not require the use of a tourniquet. The dorsal vein in the hand is used for the collection, and a needle is used to obtain the blood. The blood is collected directly from the hub of the needle.

D. The dorsal hand vein technique for neonates and infants does not require the use of a tourniquet. The dorsal vein in the hand is used for the collection, and a needle is used to obtain the blood. The blood is collected directly from the hub of the needle. (pp. 313–315)

10.

A. When a skin puncture is performed on an infant or a child, hematology specimens are collected first to minimize platelet clumping. Chemistry and blood bank specimens are collected next.

B. When a skin puncture is performed on an infant or a child, hematology specimens are collected first to minimize platelet clumping. Chemistry and blood bank specimens are collected next.

C. When a skin puncture is performed on an infant or a child, hematology specimens are collected first to minimize platelet clumping. Chemistry and blood bank specimens are collected next.

D. When a skin puncture is performed on an infant or a child, hematology specimens are collected first to minimize platelet clumping. (p. 305)

11.

A. A 10-mL blood sample taken from a premature or newborn infant is equivalent to 5 to 10 percent of the infant's total blood volume.

B. A 10-mL blood sample taken from a premature or newborn infant is equivalent to 5 to 10 percent of the infant's total blood volume.

C. A 10-mL blood sample taken from a premature or newborn infant is equivalent to 5 to 10 percent of the infant's total blood volume. (p. 304)

D. A 10-mL blood sample taken from a premature or newborn infant is equivalent to 5 to 10 percent of the infant's total blood volume.

12.

A. For pediatric skin puncture, the following equipment is needed (p. 305):

1. sterile automatic disposable pediatric safety lancet devices
2. 70 percent isopropyl alcohol swabs in sterile packages
3. sterile cotton balls or gauze sponges
4. plastic capillary collection tubes and sealer
5. microcollection containers and Unopettes
6. glass slides for smears
7. puncture-resistant sharps container
8. disposable gloves (nonlatex if child is allergic)
9. compress (towel or washcloth) to warm heel if necessary
10. marking pen
11. laboratory request slips or labels

B. For pediatric skin puncture, the following equipment is needed:

1. sterile automatic disposable pediatric safety lancet devices
2. 70 percent isopropyl alcohol swabs in sterile packages
3. sterile cotton balls or gauze sponges
4. plastic capillary collection tubes and sealer
5. microcollection containers and Unopettes
6. glass slides for smears
7. puncture-resistant sharps container
8. disposable gloves (nonlatex if child is allergic)
9. compress (towel or washcloth) to warm heel if necessary
10. marking pen
11. laboratory request slips or labels

C. For pediatric skin puncture, the following equipment is needed:

1. sterile automatic disposable pediatric safety lancet devices
2. 70 percent isopropyl alcohol swabs in sterile packages
3. sterile cotton balls or gauze sponges
4. plastic capillary collection tubes and sealer
5. microcollection containers and Unopettes
6. glass slides for smears
7. puncture-resistant sharps container
8. disposable gloves (nonlatex if child is allergic)
9. compress (towel or washcloth) to warm heel if necessary

10. marking pen
11. laboratory request slips or labels

D. For pediatric skin puncture, the following equipment is needed:

1. sterile automatic disposable pediatric safety lancet devices
2. 70 percent isopropyl alcohol swabs in sterile packages
3. sterile cotton balls or gauze sponges
4. plastic capillary collection tubes and sealer
5. microcollection containers and Unopettes
6. glass slides for smears
7. puncture-resistant sharps container
8. disposable gloves (nonlatex if child is allergic)
9. compress (towel or washcloth) to warm heel if necessary
10. marking pen
11. laboratory request slips or labels

13.

A. The total blood volume of a premature infant is calculated by multiplying the weight in kilograms by 115 mL/kg. (p. 305)

B. The total blood volume of a newborn infant is calculated by multiplying the baby's weight in kilograms by 80 to 110 mL/kg blood volume.

C. This is the blood volume calculation to be used for infants and children.

D. This is the blood volume calculation to be used for adults.

14.

A. In the United States, neonatal blood screening for phenylketonuria (PKU) and hypothyroidism is mandatory by law.

B. In the United States, neonatal blood screening for phenylketonuria (PKU) and hypothyroidism is mandatory by law. (p. 312)

C. In the United States, neonatal blood screening for phenylketonuria (PKU) and hypothyroidism is mandatory by law.

D. In the United States, neonatal blood screening for phenylketonuria (PKU) and hypothyroidism is mandatory by law.

15.

A. After blood is collected for PKU testing, the card must thoroughly dry in a horizontal position for a minimum of 3 hours.

B. After blood is collected for PKU testing, the card must thoroughly dry in a horizontal position for a minimum of 3 hours.

C. After blood is collected for PKU testing, the card must thoroughly dry in a horizontal position for a minimum of 3 hours.

D. After blood is collected for PKU testing, the card must thoroughly dry in a horizontal position for a minimum of 3 hours. (p. 312)

16.

A. When collecting blood from a saline lock on a child, the blood collector must check the patency of the line by flushing with a small amount of normal saline.

B. When collecting blood from a saline lock on a child, the blood collector must check the patency of the line by flushing with a small amount of normal saline. (p. 317)

C. When collecting blood from a saline lock on a child, the blood collector must check the patency of the line by flushing with a small amount of normal saline.

D. When collecting blood from a saline lock on a child, the blood collector must check the patency of the line by flushing with a small amount of normal saline.

17.

A. The topical anesthetic EMLA (eutectic mixture of local anesthetics), which is an emulsion of lidocaine and prilocaine, can be applied to an infant or child to alleviate pain from venipuncture.

B. The topical anesthetic EMLA (eutectic mixture of local anesthetics), which is an emulsion of lidocaine and prilocaine, can be applied to an infant or child to alleviate pain from venipuncture.

C. The topical anesthetic EMLA (eutectic mixture of local anesthetics), which is an emulsion of lidocaine

and prilocaine, can be applied to an infant or child to alleviate pain from venipuncture.

D. The topical anesthetic EMLA (eutectic mixture of local anesthetics), which is an emulsion of lidocaine and prilocaine, can be applied to an infant or child to alleviate pain from venipuncture. (p. 303)

18.

A. The anteromedial aspect or the posterior curve of the heel must not be used for a skin puncture site because a puncture at either site could injure the underlying calcaneus.

B. The preferred site for a heel stick is the medial or lateral aspect of the heel. (pp. 306–307)

C. The anteromedial aspect or the posterior curve of the heel must not be used for a skin puncture site because a puncture at either site could injure the underlying calcaneus.

D. Avoid heel sticks in an area that has previous puncture sites because such a stick could cause an infection.

19.

A. Compared with skin puncture, dorsal hand venipuncture on an infant is less stressful for the infant and the health care provider, there is less dilution of the specimen with tissue fluids, there is less hemolysis, and fewer punctures are required.

B. Compared with skin puncture, dorsal hand venipuncture on an infant is less stressful for the infant and the health care provider, there is less dilution of the specimen with tissue fluids, there is less hemolysis, and fewer punctures are required.

C. Compared with skin puncture, dorsal hand venipuncture on an infant is less stressful for the infant and the health care provider, there is less dilution of the specimen with tissue fluids, there is less hemolysis, and fewer punctures are required. (pp. 313–315)

D. Compared with skin puncture, dorsal hand venipuncture on an infant is less stressful for the infant and the health care provider, there is less dilution of the specimen with tissue fluids, there is less hemolysis, and fewer punctures are required.

CHAPTER

12 Arterial, Intravenous (IV), and Special Collection Procedures

chapter objectives

Upon completion of Chapter 12, the learner is responsible for the following:

➤ Explain the special precautions and types of equipment needed to collect capillary or arterial blood gases.

➤ Describe the equipment that is used to perform the bleeding-time test.

➤ Discuss the requirements for the glucose and lactose tolerance tests.

➤ Differentiate cannulas from fistulas.

➤ List the steps and equipment in blood culture collections.

➤ List the special requirements for collecting blood through central venous catheters (CVCs).

➤ Differentiate therapeutic phlebotomy from autologous transfusion.

➤ Describe the special precautions needed to collect blood in therapeutic drug monitoring (TDM) procedures.

➤ List the types of patient specimens that are needed for trace metal analyses.

DIRECTIONS Each of the questions or incomplete statements below is followed by four suggested answers or completions. Select **one answer** that is best in each case.

 KNOWLEDGE LEVEL = 1

1. Cleansing the venipuncture site before collection of blood culture specimens usually involves the use of:
   A. isopropyl alcohol and peroxide
   B. ethyl alcohol and peroxide
   C. povidone-iodine and peroxide
   D. povidone-iodine and alcohol

 KNOWLEDGE LEVEL = 2

2. Which of the following is the specimen of choice for testing the pH, pO_2, and pCO_2 of the blood?
   A. arterial blood
   B. venous blood
   C. heparinized plasma
   D. skin puncture blood

 KNOWLEDGE LEVEL = 1

3. Which of the following sites is *not* recommended to collect capillary blood gases?
   A. lateral posterior area of the heel
   B. lateral anterior area of the elbow
   C. the great toe
   D. the ball of the finger

 KNOWLEDGE LEVEL = 1

4. What should be the minimum volume of the capillary tube used to collect a specimen for capillary blood gas analysis?
   A. 25 μL
   B. 50 μL
   C. 100 μL
   D. 200 μL

 KNOWLEDGE LEVEL = 1

5. Which of the following supplies is *not* needed during an arterial puncture for an ABG determination?
   A. syringe
   B. tourniquet
   C. gloves
   D. lidocaine

 KNOWLEDGE LEVEL = 1

6. When blood is collected from the radial artery for an arterial blood gas collection, the needle should be inserted at an angle of no less than:
   A. 15 degrees
   B. 25 degrees
   C. 35 degrees
   D. 45 degrees

 KNOWLEDGE LEVEL = 1

7. Which of the following is the preferred site for blood collection for arterial blood gas analysis?
   A. ulnar artery
   B. femoral artery
   C. radial artery
   D. subclavian artery

 KNOWLEDGE LEVEL = 3

8. What is the rationale for performing the Allen test?
   A. to test for the possibility of edema
   B. to determine whether the patient's blood pressure is elevated

C. to determine that the radial and ulnar arteries are providing collateral circulation

D. to determine whether the oxygen concentration in the radial artery is sufficient for the blood collection

 KNOWLEDGE LEVEL = 1

9. Which of the following evacuated tubes is preferred for the collection of arterial blood gas analysis?
   A. yellow-topped evacuated tube
   B. green-topped evacuated tube
   C. light blue-topped evacuated tube
   D. no evacuated tube

 KNOWLEDGE LEVEL = 1

10. Which of the following evacuated tubes is preferred for the collection of a blood culture specimen?
    A. yellow-topped evacuated tube
    B. green-topped evacuated tube
    C. speckled-topped evacuated tube
    D. light blue-topped evacuated tube

 KNOWLEDGE LEVEL = 1

11. What is a cannula?
    A. a good source of arterial blood
    B. the fusion of a vein and an artery
    C. a tubular instrument used to gain access to venous blood
    D. an artificial shunt that provides access to arterial blood

KNOWLEDGE LEVEL = 2

12. For central venous catheter (CVC) blood collections, which of the following blood analytes should *not* be collected if heparin is infusing into the line?
    A. CPK
    B. PT
    C. ALT
    D. AST

 KNOWLEDGE LEVEL = 3

13. The bleeding-time test is used to:
    A. check for vascular abnormalities
    B. diagnose diabetes mellitus
    C. determine whether the patient's blood pressure is low
    D. access liver glycogen stores

 KNOWLEDGE LEVEL = 1

14. Which of the following tubes must be collected first?
    A. red-topped evacuated tube
    B. yellow-topped evacuated tube
    C. light blue-topped evacuated tube
    D. royal blue-topped evacuated tube

 KNOWLEDGE LEVEL = 2

15. Which of the following is used to help in the diagnosis of diabetes mellitus?
    A. ABG analysis
    B. PT
    C. TDM
    D. GTT

 KNOWLEDGE LEVEL = 1

16. *Postprandial* refers to:
    A. 2-hour fasting
    B. 12-hour fasting
    C. after eating
    D. before eating

KNOWLEDGE LEVEL = 1

17. Which of the following is the preferred gauge of a needle used for blood collection from a donor?
    A. 17
    B. 20
    C. 21
    D. 23

 KNOWLEDGE LEVEL = 1

18. The Isostat system (Wampole Laboratories, Cranbury, NJ) is a:
    A. heparin lock system within a central venous catheter
    B. bleeding-time system
    C. special blood culture tube system
    D. special arterial blood gas syringe

 KNOWLEDGE LEVEL = 3

19. To obtain the blood trough level for a medication, the patient's blood should be collected:
    A. immediately after administration of the medication
    B. immediately before administration of the medication
    C. 2 hours before administration of the medication
    D. 2 hours after administration of the medication

 KNOWLEDGE LEVEL = 1

20. Which of the following tests requires numerous blood collections?
    A. arterial blood gas analysis
    B. GTT
    C. bleeding-time test
    D. drug screening

 KNOWLEDGE LEVEL = 1

21. Which of the following procedures requires blood collection for trough and peak level determinations?
    A. skin test for allergies
    B. therapeutic drug monitoring
    C. blood collection through CVCs
    D. sweat chloride procedure

 KNOWLEDGE LEVEL = 2

22. Which of the following procedures helps to reduce potential scarring from the Surgicutt bleeding-time test?
    A. Apply a butterfly-type bandage to the incision site.
    B. Provide a small stitch to the incision site.
    C. Apply gauze and tape to the incision site.
    D. Apply a small piece of moleskin to the incision site.

 KNOWLEDGE LEVEL = 1

23. For the Surgicutt bleeding-time test, the blood pressure cuff must be inflated on the patient's upper arm to
    A. 20 mm Hg
    B. 30 mm Hg
    C. 40 mm Hg
    D. 60 mm Hg

 KNOWLEDGE LEVEL = 1

24. The health care worker's thumb should not be used for palpating arteries in the arterial puncture procedure because the thumb:
    A. is usually dirty
    B. has less sensitivity than the other fingers
    C. has a pulse that may be confused with the patient's pulse
    D. has more neurons for touching, which interfere in the process of finding the patient's pulse

KNOWLEDGE LEVEL = 2

25. Blood gas analysis includes testing for:
    A. pH, pH$_2$O, and pCO$_2$
    B. pH, pO$_2$, and pCO$_2$
    C. pH$_2$O, pCO$_2$, and pO$_2$
    D. pH$_2$O, pH, and pO$_2$

 KNOWLEDGE LEVEL = 3

26. If the patient's bleeding time is longer than the normal limits, which of the following laboratory tests may be needed?
    A. alkaline phosphatase level
    B. acid phosphatase level
    C. platelet count
    D. blood urea nitrogen result

 KNOWLEDGE LEVEL = 2

27. Which of the following procedures requires 10 mL of normal saline and two or three 20-mL disposable syringes?
    A. sweat chloride procedure
    B. skin test for allergies
    C. blood collection from a blood donor
    D. blood collection through CVCs

 KNOWLEDGE LEVEL = 3

28. Which of the following is a coagulopathy?
    A. diabetes mellitus
    B. von Gierke's disease
    C. von Willebrand's disease
    D. diabetes insipidus

 KNOWLEDGE LEVEL = 3

29. Which of the following guidelines must the patient abide by to properly prepare himself or herself for the GTT?

A. The patient's carbohydrate intake must not exceed 20 g per day for 3 days before the GTT.
B. The patient must not eat anything for 12 hours before the GTT but should not fast for more than 14 hours before the test.
C. The patient should take corticosteroids 2 days before the GTT
D. The patient should vigorously exercise within 8 to 12 hours before the GTT.

 KNOWLEDGE LEVEL = 3

30. Which of the following drugs has a shorter half-life and therefore requires exact timing in blood collection for its therapeutic level?
    A. procainamide
    B. phenobarbital
    C. digoxin
    D. digitoxin

 KNOWLEDGE LEVEL = 1

31. Normally, after an adult patient ingests the 75 or 100 g of glucose in the glucose tolerance test, the glucose level should return to normal within how many minutes?
    A. 30
    B. 60
    C. 120
    D. 180

 KNOWLEDGE LEVEL = 2

32. Before a blood donation, the phlebotomist must always check the blood donor's:
    A. blood glucose value
    B. hematocrit or hemoglobin value
    C. urine glucose value
    D. WBC count

KNOWLEDGE LEVEL = 2

33. An autologous transfusion is used to prevent which of the following possibilities?
    A. Polycythemia will develop in the transfused patient.
    B. Antigens will form in the transfused patient.
    C. Antibodies will form in the transfused patient.
    D. The transfused patient will develop diabetes mellitus.

 KNOWLEDGE LEVEL = 3

34. During a glucose tolerance test, which procedure is acceptable?
    A. A standard amount of glucose drink is given to the patient, then a fasting blood collection is performed.
    B. The patient should be encouraged to drink water throughout the procedure.
    C. The patient is allowed to chew sugarless gum.
    D. All the patient's specimens are timed from the fasting collection.

 KNOWLEDGE LEVEL = 2

35. Which of the following is a milk sugar that sometimes cannot be digested by healthy individuals?
    A. glucose
    B. glucagon
    C. lactose
    D. lactate

 KNOWLEDGE LEVEL = 3

36. Which of the following is the correct protocol in the collection of blood for blood cultures?

A. palpating the venipuncture site after the site has been prepared without first cleaning the chemically cleaned gloved finger
B. injecting air into the anaerobic bottle
C. inoculating the anaerobic bottle last
D. wiping the iodine from the tops of the bottles with alcohol

 KNOWLEDGE LEVEL = 2

37. The following materials and/or supplies are needed for the Surgicutt procedure except:
    A. blood pressure cuff
    B. butterfly-type bandage
    C. disposable gloves
    D. vacuum blood collection tube with EDTA

 KNOWLEDGE LEVEL = 1

38. Figure 12.1 shows swabbing of the arm in concentric circles in preparation of collecting blood for:
    A. therapeutic drug monitoring
    B. toxicology studies
    C. blood donation
    D. lactose tolerance test

 KNOWLEDGE LEVEL = 1

39. A tubular instrument that is used in kidney patients to gain access to venous blood for dialysis or blood collection is referred to as a:
    A. CVC
    B. cannula
    C. fistula
    D. venous isolator

FIGURE 12.1.

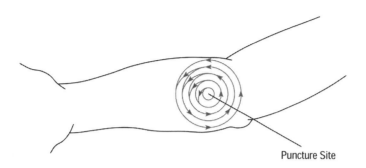

Puncture Site

KNOWLEDGE LEVEL = 2

40. Therapeutic phlebotomy is used in the treatment of:
    A. megaloblastic anemia
    B. polycythemia
    C. chronic anemia
    D. iron-deficiency anemia

KNOWLEDGE LEVEL = 1

41. To help minimize the incidence of dizziness, fainting, or other reactions to blood loss, blood donors are encouraged to eat within how many hours of donating blood?
    A. 9
    B. 8
    C. 7
    D. 6

KNOWLEDGE LEVEL = 2

42. Which of the following items is *not* usually kept on file for every blood donor indefinitely?
    A. age
    B. a written consent form signed by the donor
    C. a record of reason for deferrals
    D. a written consent form signed by the donor's parent

KNOWLEDGE LEVEL = 1

43. For a donor to donate blood, his or her oral temperature must not exceed:
    A. 35°C
    B. 37.5°C
    C. 38.7°C
    D. 39.5°F

KNOWLEDGE LEVEL = 1

44. For the brief physical examination that is required to determine whether a blood donor is in generally good health, the donor's systolic blood pressure should measure:
    A. 50 to 100 mm Hg
    B. 60 to 110 mm Hg
    C. 90 to 180 mm Hg
    D. 100 to 190 mm Hg

 KNOWLEDGE LEVEL = 3

45. A false-negative blood culture is more likely to occur if:
    A. iodine is not wiped from the tops of the blood culture tubes
    B. the indwelling catheter is used to obtain the culture specimen
    C. too much blood is used for the culture
    D. the health care worker palpates the venipuncture site after the site has been prepared without first cleaning the gloved finger.

 KNOWLEDGE LEVEL = 2

46. Blood glucose levels are measured for patients undergoing:
    A. Allen test
    B. blood gas analysis
    C. lactose tolerance test
    D. therapeutic phlebotomy

 KNOWLEDGE LEVEL = 3

47. Which of the following can lead to deferral of a person from blood donation?
    A. weighs 110 pounds
    B. has an oral temperature of 37°C
    C. has a hematocrit value of 36%
    D. has a pulse rate of 70 beats per minute

 KNOWLEDGE LEVEL = 2

48. Which of the following can lead to deferral of a person from blood donation? The potential donor has:
    A. poison ivy rash on his or her arms
    B. purulent skin lesions on his or her arms
    C. psoriasis skin lesions on his or her arms
    D. acne skin lesions on his or her arms

 KNOWLEDGE LEVEL = 2

49. If a potential donor is allergic to iodine, then in venipuncture site preparation for blood donation, the phlebotomist should use which of the following?
    A. 1% PVP without iodine
    B. alcohol only
    C. acetone alcohol
    D. 0.75% PVP-iodine

 KNOWLEDGE LEVEL = 3

50. An artificial shunt in which the vein and artery have been fused through surgery is usually found in:
    A. cardiac patients
    B. kidney dialysis patients
    C. patients with liver disease
    D. patients with arm amputations

 KNOWLEDGE LEVEL = 2

51. Which of the following laboratory tests requires the use of a specially prepared acid-washed plastic syringe when the test specimen is collected in a syringe?
    A. blood culture
    B. blood gas
    C. glucose
    D. trace metals

FIGURE 12.2.

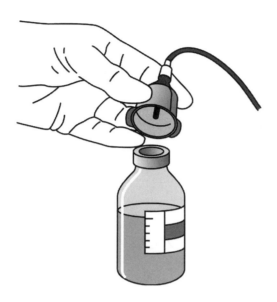

 KNOWLEDGE LEVEL = 1

52. Which of the following is for bleeding-time tests?
    A. Isostat system
    B. Simplate R
    C. BACTEC PLUS
    D. Allen test

 KNOWLEDGE LEVEL = 3

53. When using the blood culture collection device shown in Figure 12.2, which of the following is correct?
    A. The blood is transferred to the aerobic vial first.
    B. The blood is transferred to the anaerobic vial first.
    C. If only 3 mL of blood can be collected, the entire amount should be placed in the anaerobic vial.
    D. The blood is usually transferred directly from a CVC line.

 KNOWLEDGE LEVEL = 3

54. As a phlebotomist, you have just completed the collection of a GTT on a 28-year-old female patient who asks you whether it is okay that she has eaten only meat and eggs for the past week before this test. What do you tell her?
    A. Yes, the GTT results will not be affected.
    B. No, the GTT results will be falsely affected because she should have been on the only meat and eggs diet for 2 weeks.
    C. No, the GTT results will be falsely affected because the test is based on a person having a carbohydrate intake that must be at least 150 grams per day for 14 days before the GTT.
    D. No, the GTT results will be falsely affected because the test is based on a person having a carbohydrate intake that must be at least 150 grams per day for 3 days before the GTT.

KNOWLEDGE LEVEL = 2

55. The purpose of the GTT is to test the patient's:
    A. insulin-releasing mechanism
    B. lactose-releasing mechanism
    C. thyroid function
    D. liver function

 KNOWLEDGE LEVEL = 2

56. A false-positive blood culture is more likely to occur if:
    A. iodine is not wiped from the tops of the blood culture tubes
    B. too much blood is used for the culture
    C. too little blood is used for the culture
    D. povidone-iodine solution is used to clean the venipuncture site but not the cleaned gloved palpating finger

 KNOWLEDGE LEVEL = 1

57. For blood culture collections, the most appropriate needle gauge size to use is:
    A. 17-gauge
    B. 18-gauge
    C. 19-gauge
    D. 22-gauge

 KNOWLEDGE LEVEL = 2

58. Blood cultures are often collected from patients who have:
    A. FUO
    B. FKO
    C. rabies
    D. Von Willebrand's disease

 KNOWLEDGE LEVEL = 1

59. One percent lidocaine is used in:
    A. blood culture collection
    B. arterial blood gas collection
    C. therapeutic phlebotomy
    D. bleeding-time test

 KNOWLEDGE LEVEL = 1

60. Which of the following procedures does *not* require cleansing the blood collection site with povidone-iodine solution?
    A. therapeutic drug monitoring collection
    B. arterial blood gas collection
    C. blood culture collection
    D. blood donation collection

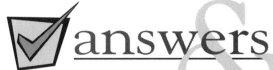

answers & rationales

1.

A. Cleansing the venipuncture site before collection of blood culture specimens usually involves the use of povidone-iodine and alcohol.

B. Cleansing the venipuncture site before collection of blood culture specimens usually involves the use of povidone-iodine and alcohol.

C. Cleansing the venipuncture site before collection of blood culture specimens usually involves the use of povidone-iodine and alcohol.

D. Cleansing the venipuncture site before collection of blood culture specimens usually involves the use of povidone-iodine and alcohol. (pp. 334–336)

2.

A. Arterial blood is the specimen of choice for testing the pH, pO_2, and pCO_2 of the blood. Arterial blood is used rather than venous blood because arterial blood has the same composition throughout the body tissues, whereas venous blood has various compositions relative to metabolic activities in body tissues. (p. 324)

B. Arterial blood is the specimen of choice for testing the pH, pO_2, and pCO_2 of the blood. Arterial blood is used rather than venous blood because arterial blood has the same composition throughout the body tissues, whereas venous blood has various compositions relative to metabolic activities in body tissues.

C. Arterial blood is the specimen of choice for testing the pH, pO_2, and pCO_2 of the blood. Arterial blood is used rather than venous blood because arterial blood has the same composition throughout the body tissues, whereas venous blood has various compositions relative to metabolic activities in body tissues.

D. Arterial blood is the specimen of choice for testing the pH, pO_2, and pCO_2 of the blood. Arterial blood is used rather than venous blood because arterial blood has the same composition throughout the body tissues, whereas venous blood has various compositions relative to metabolic activities in body tissues.

3.

A. Blood for capillary blood gas analysis is collected from the same areas of the body as other capillary samples, such as the lateral posterior area of the heel, the great toe, or the ball of the finger.

B. Blood for capillary blood gas analysis is collected from the same areas of the body as other capillary samples, such as the lateral posterior area of the heel, the great toe, or the ball of the finger. (p. 330)

C. Blood for capillary blood gas analysis is collected from the same areas of the body as other capillary samples, such as the lateral posterior area of the heel, the great toe, or the ball of the finger.

D. Blood for capillary blood gas analysis is collected from the same areas of the body as other capillary samples, such as the lateral posterior area of the heel, the great toe, or the ball of the finger.

4.

A. A heparinized capillary tube with a volume of at least 100 μL should be used to collect a specimen for capillary blood gas analysis.

B. A heparinized capillary tube with a volume of at least 100 μL should be used to collect a specimen for capillary blood gas analysis.

C. A heparinized capillary tube with a volume of at least 100 μL should be used to collect a specimen for capillary blood gas analysis. (p. 330)

D. A heparinized capillary tube with a volume of at least 100 μL should be used to collect a specimen for capillary blood gas analysis.

5.

A. As in venipuncture, a syringe with a needle is used to collect the blood.

B. No tourniquet is required because the artery has its own strong blood pressure. (p. 329)

C. As in any blood collection procedure, gloves are required for the procedure.

D. Lidocaine, in 1/2 to 1 percent, is needed to numb the site.

6.

A. The health care worker should pierce the pulsating artery at a high angle, usually no less than 45 degrees.

B. The health care worker should pierce the pulsating artery at a high angle, usually no less than 45 degrees.

C. The health care worker should pierce the pulsating artery at a high angle, usually no less than 45 degrees.

D. The health care worker should pierce the pulsating artery at a high angle, usually no less than 45 degrees. (p. 329)

7.

A. When an arterial blood gas analysis is ordered, the health care worker should palpate the radial artery in the radial sulcus of the forearm, since the radial artery in the patient's nondominant hand is usually the best choice.

B. When an arterial blood gas analysis is ordered, the health care worker should palpate the radial artery in the radial sulcus of the forearm, since the radial artery in the patient's nondominant hand is usually the best choice.

C. When an arterial blood gas analysis is ordered, the health care worker should palpate the radial artery in the radial sulcus of the forearm, since the radial artery in the patient's nondominant hand is usually the best choice. (p. 327)

D. When an arterial blood gas analysis is ordered, the health care worker should palpate the radial artery in the radial sulcus of the forearm, since the radial artery in the patient's nondominant hand is usually the best choice.

8.

A. To use the radial artery for blood collection for arterial blood gas analysis, the health care provider must first perform the Allen test to make certain that the ulnar and radial arteries are providing collateral circulation.

B. To use the radial artery for blood collection for arterial blood gas analysis, the health care provider must first perform the Allen test to make certain that the ulnar and radial arteries are providing collateral circulation.

C. To use the radial artery for blood collection for arterial blood gas analysis, the health care provider must first perform the Allen test to make certain that the ulnar and radial arteries are providing collateral circulation. (p. 324)

D. To use the radial artery for blood collection for arterial blood gas analysis, the health care provider must first perform the Allen test to make certain that the ulnar and radial arteries are providing collateral circulation.

9.

A. For the radial artery blood gas collection, a syringe is used, since little or no suction is needed because the blood pulsates and flows quickly into the syringe under its own pressure.

B. For the radial artery blood gas collection, a syringe is used, since little or no suction is needed because the blood pulsates and flows quickly into the syringe under its own pressure.

C. For the radial artery blood gas collection, a syringe is used, since little or no suction is needed because the blood pulsates and flows quickly into the syringe under its own pressure.

D. For the radial artery blood gas collection, a syringe is used, since little or no suction is needed because the blood pulsates and flows quickly into the syringe under its own pressure. (p. 329)

10.

A. Blood culture specimens need to be collected in SPS (yellow-topped) evacuated tubes. (pp. 335, 338)

B. Blood culture specimens need to be collected in SPS (yellow-topped) evacuated tubes.

C. Blood culture specimens need to be collected in SPS (yellow-topped) evacuated tubes.

D. Blood culture specimens need to be collected in SPS (yellow-topped) evacuated tubes.

11.

A. A cannula is a tubular instrument that is used in patients with kidney disease to gain access to venous blood for dialysis or blood collections.

B. A cannula is a tubular instrument that is used in patients with kidney disease to gain access to venous blood for dialysis or blood collections.

C. A cannula is a tubular instrument that is used in patients with kidney disease to gain access to venous blood for dialysis or blood collections. (p. 351)

D. A cannula is a tubular instrument that is used in patients with kidney disease to gain access to venous blood for dialysis or blood collections.

12.

A. The coagulation tests, protime (PT) and partial thromboplastin time (PTT), should not be performed on blood specimens obtained from CVCs into which heparin is infusing, since heparin will erroneously alter the PT and PTT test results.

B. The coagulation tests, protime (PT) and partial thromboplastin time (PTT), should not be performed on blood specimens obtained from CVCs into which heparin is infusing, since heparin will erroneously alter the PT and PTT test results. (p. 350)

C. The coagulation tests, protime (PT) and partial thromboplastin time (PTT), should not be performed on blood specimens obtained from CVCs into which heparin is infusing, since heparin will erroneously alter the PT and PTT test results.

D. The coagulation tests, protime (PT) and partial thromboplastin time (PTT), should not be performed on blood specimens obtained from CVCs into which heparin is infusing, since heparin will erroneously alter the PT and PTT test results.

13.

A. The bleeding-time test is a useful tool for testing platelet plug formation in the capillaries to diagnose coagulopathies or problems in hemostasis, such as vascular abnormalities. (p. 331)

B. The bleeding-time test is a useful tool for testing platelet plug formation in the capillaries to diagnose coagulopathies or problems in hemostasis, such as vascular abnormalities.

C. The bleeding-time test is a useful tool for testing platelet plug formation in the capillaries to diagnose coagulopathies or problems in hemostasis, such as vascular abnormalities.

D. The bleeding-time test is a useful tool for testing platelet plug formation in the capillaries to diagnose coagulopathies or problems in hemostasis, such as vascular abnormalities.

14.

A. If blood culture collections are ordered with other laboratory tests, blood culture specimens (i.e., collected in the SPS-yellow-topped evacuated tube) must be collected first to avoid contamination of the blood specimen.

B. If blood culture collections are ordered with other laboratory tests, blood culture specimens (i.e., collected in the SPS-yellow-topped evacuated tube) must be collected first to avoid contamination of the blood specimen. (p. 338)

C. If blood culture collections are ordered with other laboratory tests, blood culture specimens (i.e., collected in the SPS-yellow-topped evacuated tube) must be collected first to avoid contamination of the blood specimen.

D. If blood culture collections are ordered with other laboratory tests, blood culture specimens (i.e., collected in the SPS-yellow-topped evacuated tube) must be collected first to avoid contamination of the blood specimen.

15.

A. The arterial blood gas (ABG) analysis is used to detect respiratory and acid-base imbalances in patients.

B. The protime (PT) is a coagulation test used to detect abnormal clotting in patients.

C. Therapeutic drug monitoring (TDM) is used to monitor the serum concentration of certain drugs such as anticonvulsant drugs, tricyclic antidepressants, and digoxin.

D. The glucose tolerance test (GTT) can be an effective diagnostic tool for patients who have symptoms suggesting problems in carbohydrate metabolism. (p. 341)

16.

A. *Postprandial* means "after eating."

B. *Postprandial* means "after eating."

C. *Postprandial* means "after eating." (p. 344)

D. *Postprandial* means "after eating."

17.

A. A 17-gauge thin-walled needle is the preferred needle for blood collection from a donor. The internal diameter of a 17-gauge needle prevents hemolysis of the red blood cells. (p. 354)

B. A 17-gauge thin-walled needle is the preferred needle for blood collection from a donor. The internal diameter of a 17-gauge needle prevents hemolysis of the red blood cells.

C. A 17-gauge thin-walled needle is the preferred needle for blood collection from a donor. The internal diameter of a 17-gauge needle prevents hemolysis of the red blood cells.

D. A 17-gauge thin-walled needle is the preferred needle for blood collection from a donor. The internal diameter of a 17-gauge needle prevents hemolysis of the red blood cells.

18.

A. The Isostat system is a special blood culture tube system that can provide faster microbial diagnostic test results; and it helps safeguard the phlebotomist since the reagents in the Isolator tube inactivate HIV within a 60-minute transport and processing time.

B. The Isostat system is a special blood culture tube system that can provide faster microbial diagnostic test results; and it helps safeguard the phlebotomist since the reagents in the Isolator tube inactivate HIV within a 60-minute transport and processing time.

C. The Isostat system is a special blood culture tube system that can provide faster microbial diagnostic test results; and it helps safeguard the phlebotomist since the reagents in the Isolator tube inactivate HIV within a 60-minute transport and processing time. (pp. 339–340)

D. The Isostat system is a special blood culture tube system that can provide faster microbial diagnostic test results; and it helps safeguard the phlebotomist since the reagents in the Isolator tube inactivate HIV within a 60-minute transport and processing time.

19.

A. To obtain the blood trough level for a medication, the patient's blood should be collected immediately before the administration of the medication. The trough level is the lowest concentration in the patient's serum.

B. To obtain the blood trough level for a medication, the patient's blood should be collected immediately before the administration of the medication. The trough level is the lowest concentration in the patient's serum. (p. 345)

C. To obtain the blood trough level for a medication, the patient's blood should be collected immediately before the administration of the medication. The trough level is the lowest concentration in the patient's serum.

D. To obtain the blood trough level for a medication, the patient's blood should be collected immediately before the administration of the medication. The trough level is the lowest concentration in the patient's serum.

20.

A. The arterial blood gas analysis requires only one arterial blood collection.

B. The glucose tolerance test (GTT) is performed by obtaining fasting blood and urine specimens, giving the fasting patient a standard load of glucose, and obtaining subsequent blood and urine specimens at intervals, usually during a 5-hour period. (p. 341)

C. The bleeding-time test requires only one blood collection.

D. Drug screening usually requires a urine specimen or one blood collection.

21.

A. So that physicians can adequately evaluate the appropriate dosage levels of many drugs, the collection and evaluation of specimens for trough and peak levels are necessary in therapeutic drug monitoring.

B. So that physicians can adequately evaluate the appropriate dosage levels of many drugs, the collection and evaluation of specimens for trough and peak levels are necessary in therapeutic drug monitoring. (pp. 345–346)

C. So that physicians can adequately evaluate the appropriate dosage levels of many drugs, the collection and evaluation of specimens for trough and peak levels are necessary in therapeutic drug monitoring.

D. So that physicians can adequately evaluate the appropriate dosage levels of many drugs, the collection and evaluation of specimens for trough and peak levels are necessary in therapeutic drug monitoring.

22.

A. Applying a butterfly-type bandage to the incision area for a 24-hour period can reduce the scarring that may result from a Surgicutt bleeding-time test. (pp. 331–332)

B. Applying a butterfly-type bandage to the incision area for a 24-hour period can reduce the scarring that may result from a Surgicutt bleeding-time test.

C. Applying a butterfly-type bandage to the incision area for a 24-hour period can reduce the scarring that may result from a Surgicutt bleeding-time test.

D. Applying a butterfly-type bandage to the incision area for a 24-hour period can reduce the scarring that may result from a Surgicutt bleeding-time test.

23.

A. For the Surgicutt bleeding-time test, the blood pressure cuff must be inflated on the patient's upper arm to 40 mm Hg.

B. For the Surgicutt bleeding-time test, the blood pressure cuff must be inflated on the patient's upper arm to 40 mm Hg.

C. For the Surgicutt bleeding-time test, the blood pressure cuff must be inflated on the patient's upper arm to 40 mm Hg. (p. 332)

D. For the Surgicutt bleeding-time test, the blood pressure cuff must be inflated on the patient's upper arm to 40 mm Hg.

24.

A. The health care provider's thumb should not be used for palpating arteries in the arterial puncture procedure because the thumb has a pulse that may be confused with the patient's pulse.

B. The health care provider's thumb should not be used for palpating arteries in the arterial puncture procedure because the thumb has a pulse that may be confused with the patient's pulse.

C. The health care provider's thumb should not be used for palpating arteries in the arterial puncture procedure because the thumb has a pulse that may be confused with the patient's pulse. (p. 327)

D. The health care provider's thumb should not be used for palpating arteries in the arterial puncture procedure because the thumb has a pulse that may be confused with the patient's pulse.

25.

A. Blood gas analyses includes testing for pH, pO_2, and pCO_2. These tests provide useful information about the respiratory status and the acid-base balance in patients with pulmonary disease or other disorders.

B. Blood gas analyses includes testing for pH, pO_2, and pCO_2. These tests provide useful information about the respiratory status and the acid-base balance in patients with pulmonary disease or other disorders. (pp. 330, 188)

C. Blood gas analyses includes testing for pH, pO_2, and pCO_2. These tests provide useful information about the respiratory status and the acid-base balance in patients with pulmonary disease or other disorders.

D. Blood gas analyses includes testing for pH, pO_2, and pCO_2. These tests provide useful information about the respiratory status and the acid-base balance in patients with pulmonary disease or other disorders.

26.

A. The alkaline phosphatase level is an enzyme used to evaluate bone activity, not coagulation problems. A prolonged bleeding time may indicate the need for further coagulation testing, such as a platelet count.

B. The acid phosphatase level is an enzyme assay used to evaluate prostate activity, not coagulation problems. A prolonged bleeding time may indicate the need for further coagulation testing, such as a platelet count.

C. A prolonged bleeding time may indicate the need for further coagulation testing, such as a platelet count. (pp. 331–333)

D. Blood urea nitrogen (BUN) test results provide information on kidney function, not coagulation problems as in the bleeding time assay.

27.

A. Two or three 20-mL disposable syringes and 10 mL of normal saline are needed to collect blood through central venous catheters.

B. Two or three 20-mL disposable syringes and 10 mL of normal saline are needed to collect blood through central venous catheters.

C. Two or three 20-mL disposable syringes and 10 mL of normal saline are needed to collect blood through central venous catheters.

D. Two or three 20-mL disposable syringes and 10 mL of normal saline are needed to collect blood through central venous catheters. (p. 348)

28.

A. Diabetes mellitus is a systemic disease due to abnormalities of glucose metabolism.

B. Von Gierke's disease is a genetic disorder in which the afflicted person's liver cannot convert glycogen to glucose.

C. The bleeding-time test is a useful tool for testing platelet plug formation in the capillaries and is used with other coagulation tests for testing coagulopathies such as von Willebrand's disease. (p. 331)

D. Diabetes insipidus is a disorder in which the afflicted person has decreased or lack of antidiuretic hormone (ADH), leading to excessive urination.

29.

A. The patient needs to follow these guidelines to prepare for the GTT: (1) the patient's carbohydrate intake must be at least 150 grams per day for 3 days before the GTT, (2) the patient should not eat anything for 12 hours before the GTT but should not fast for more than 14 hours before the test, (3) the patient should avoid all possible medications, including corticosteroids, because they will interfere in the GTT, and (4) the patient should avoid exercise for 12 hours before the GTT.

B. The patient needs to follow these guidelines to prepare for the GTT: (1) the patient's carbohydrate intake must be at least 150 grams per day for 3 days before the GTT, (2) the patient should not eat anything for 12 hours before the GTT but should not fast for more than 14 hours before the test, (3) the patient should avoid all possible medications, including corticosteroids, because they will interfere in the GTT, and (4) the patient should avoid exercise for 12 hours before the GTT. (p. 342)

C. The patient needs to follow these guidelines to prepare for the GTT: (1) the patient's carbohydrate intake must be at least 150 grams per day for 3 days before the GTT, (2) the patient should not eat anything for 12 hours before the GTT but should not fast for more than 14 hours before the test, (3) the patient should avoid all possible medications, including corticosteroids, because they will interfere in the GTT, and (4) the patient should avoid exercise for 12 hours before the GTT.

D. The patient needs to follow these guidelines to prepare for the GTT: (1) the patient's carbohydrate intake must be at least 150 grams per day for 3 days before the GTT, (2) the patient should not eat anything for 12 hours before the GTT but should not fast for more than 14 hours before the test, (3) the patient should avoid all possible medications, including corticosteroids, because they will interfere in the GTT, and (4) the patient should avoid exercise for 12 hours before the GTT.

30.

A. The time of collection is much more critical for drugs with shorter half-lives (e.g., gentamicin, tobramycin, and procainamide) than for those with longer half-lives (i.e., phenobarbital, digoxin, and digitoxin). (p. 346)

B. The time of collection is much more critical for drugs with shorter half-lives (e.g., gentamicin, tobramycin, and procainamide) than for those with longer half-lives (i.e., phenobarbital, digoxin, and digitoxin).

C. The time of collection is much more critical for drugs with shorter half-lives (e.g., gentamicin, tobramycin, and procainamide) than for those with longer half-lives (i.e., phenobarbital, digoxin, and digitoxin).

D. The time of collection is much more critical for drugs with shorter half-lives (e.g., gentamicin, tobramycin, and procainamide) than for those with longer half-lives (i.e., phenobarbital, digoxin, and digitoxin).

31.

A. Normally, after an adult patient ingests the 75 or 100 g of glucose in the glucose tolerance test (GTT), the glucose level should return to normal within 2 hours.

B. Normally, after an adult patient ingests the 75 or 100 g of glucose in the glucose tolerance test (GTT), the glucose level should return to normal within 2 hours.

C. Normally, after an adult patient ingests the 75 or 100 g of glucose in the glucose tolerance test (GTT), the glucose level should return to normal within 2 hours. (pp. 341–344)

D. Normally, after an adult patient ingests the 75 or 100 g of glucose in the glucose tolerance test (GTT), the glucose level should return to normal within 2 hours.

32.

A. The blood bank phlebotomist must check the blood donor's hematocrit or hemoglobin value before the blood donation, and it must be no less than 12.5g/dL.

B. The blood bank phlebotomist must check the blood donor's hematocrit or hemoglobin value before the blood donation, and it must be no less than 12.5g/dL. (p. 353)

C. The blood bank phlebotomist must check the blood donor's hematocrit or hemoglobin value before the blood donation, and it must be no less than 12.5g/dL.

D. The blood bank phlebotomist must check the blood donor's hematocrit or hemoglobin value before the blood donation, and it must be no less than 12.5g/dL.

33.

A. The autologous transfusion prevents transfusion-transmitted infectious diseases (e.g., hepatitis C) and eliminates the formation of antibodies in the transfused patient.

B. The autologous transfusion prevents transfusion-transmitted infectious diseases (e.g., hepatitis C) and eliminates the formation of antibodies in the transfused patient.

C. The autologous transfusion prevents transfusion-transmitted infectious diseases (e.g., hepatitis C) and eliminates the formation of antibodies in the transfused patient. (p. 361)

D. The autologous transfusion prevents transfusion-transmitted infectious diseases (e.g., hepatitis C) and eliminates the formation of antibodies in the transfused patient.

34.

A. A fasting blood collection is performed in the GTT, and then a standard amount of glucose drink is given to the patient.

B. During the glucose tolerance test (GTT), the patient is required to have numerous urine collections to test for glucose. Therefore it is imperative for the patient to drink water during the GTT. However, other liquids have to be avoided, since they will interfere in the test results. (p. 341)

C. Sugarless gum must be avoided in the GTT procedure, since it can stimulate digestion and interfere in the test results.

D. All the patient's specimens in the GTT are timed from the minute the patient finishes drinking the glucose solution.

35.

A. Some otherwise healthy individuals experience difficulty in digesting lactose, a milk sugar. They appear to lack a mucosal lactase enzyme that breaks down the lactose into the simple sugars glucose and galactose.

B. Some otherwise healthy individuals experience difficulty in digesting lactose, a milk sugar. They appear to lack a mucosal lactase enzyme that breaks down the lactose into the simple sugars glucose and galactose.

C. Some otherwise healthy individuals experience difficulty in digesting lactose, a milk sugar. They appear to lack a mucosal lactase enzyme that breaks down the lactose into the simple sugars glucose and galactose. (p. 344)

D. Some otherwise healthy individuals experience difficulty in digesting lactose, a milk sugar. They appear to lack a mucosal lactase enzyme that breaks down the lactose into the simple sugars glucose and galactose.

36.

A. Iodine may interfere in the blood culture results and therefore must be wiped from the tops of the collection bottles with alcohol.

B. Iodine may interfere in the blood culture results and therefore must be wiped from the tops of the collection bottles with alcohol.

C. Iodine may interfere in the blood culture results and therefore must be wiped from the tops of the collection bottles with alcohol.

D. Iodine may interfere in the blood culture results and therefore must be wiped from the tops of the collection bottles with alcohol. (pp. 334–336)

37.

A. A blood pressure cuff (sphygmomanometer), a butterfly-type bandage, and disposable gloves are needed for the Surgicutt procedure. It is a bleeding time procedure, and therefore vacuum blood collection tubes are not required.

B. A blood pressure cuff (sphygmomanometer), a butterfly-type bandage, and disposable gloves are needed for the Surgicutt procedure. It is a bleeding time procedure, and therefore vacuum blood collection tubes are not required.

C. A blood pressure cuff (sphygmomanometer), a butterfly-type bandage, and disposable gloves are needed for the Surgicutt procedure. It is a bleeding time procedure, and therefore vacuum blood collection tubes are not required.

D. A blood pressure cuff (sphygmomanometer), a butterfly-type bandage, and disposable gloves are needed for the Surgicutt procedure. It is a bleeding time procedure, and therefore vacuum blood collection tubes are not required. (pp. 331–333)

38.

A. For therapeutic drug-monitoring collections, a regular cleansing procedure of the venipuncture site is needed.

B. Blood collected for toxicology studies requires a regular cleansing procedure. However, isopropyl alcohol cannot be used as the cleansing solution if blood alcohol levels are being requested.

C. For blood donations, if the donor is not allergic to iodine, a 0.75% PVP-iodine scrub solution is used to scrub the intended phlebotomy site in concentric circles in a 3-inch-diameter area around the venipuncture site. A green soap scrub is used for donors who are allergic to iodine. (p. 367)

D. The lactose tolerance test requires only the usual cleansing procedure for venipuncture collections.

39.

A. CVC is the acronym for central venous catheter which is also called an intravenous (IV) line.

B. A cannula is a tubular instrument that is used in kidney patients to gain access to venous blood for dialysis or blood collection. (p. 351)

C. A fistula is an artificial shunt in which the vein and artery have been fused through surgery.

D. A cannula is a tubular instrument that is used in kidney patients to gain access to venous blood for dialysis or blood collection.

40.

A. Therapeutic phlebotomy is the intentional removal of blood in conditions in which there is an excessive production of blood cells, as in polycythemia.

B. Therapeutic phlebotomy is the intentional removal of blood in conditions in which there is an excessive production of blood cells, as in polycythemia. (p. 361)

C. Therapeutic phlebotomy is the intentional removal of blood in conditions in which there is an excessive production of blood cells, as in polycythemia.

D. Therapeutic phlebotomy is the intentional removal of blood in conditions in which there is an excessive production of blood cells, as in polycythemia.

41.

A. To help minimize the incidence of dizziness, fainting, or other reactions to blood loss, blood donors are encouraged to eat within 4 to 6 hours of donating blood.

B. To help minimize the incidence of dizziness, fainting, or other reactions to blood loss, blood donors are encouraged to eat within 4 to 6 hours of donating blood.

C. To help minimize the incidence of dizziness, fainting, or other reactions to blood loss, blood donors are encouraged to eat within 4 to 6 hours of donating blood.

D. To help minimize the incidence of dizziness, fainting, or other reactions to blood loss, blood donors are encouraged to eat within 4 to 6 hours of donating blood. (p. 356)

42.

A. Several items must be kept on file on every donor indefinitely, including age, name, date of birth, a written consent form signed by the donor, and a record of reason for deferrals. The donor, not the donor's parents, consents to his or her own blood collection.

B. Several items must be kept on file on every donor indefinitely, including age, name, date of birth, a written consent form signed by the donor, and a record of reason for deferrals. The donor, not the donor's parents, consents to his or her own blood collection.

C. Several items must be kept on file on every donor indefinitely, including age, name, date of birth, a written consent form signed by the donor, and a record of reason for deferrals. The donor, not the donor's parents, consents to his or her own blood collection.

D. Several items must be kept on file on every donor indefinitely, including age, name, date of birth, a written consent form signed by the donor, and a record of reason for deferrals. The donor, not the donor's parents, consents to his or her own blood collection. (pp. 352–353)

43.

A. The donor's oral temperature must not exceed 37.5°C (99.5°F).

B. The donor's oral temperature must not exceed 37.5°C (99.5°F). (p. 353)

C. The donor's oral temperature must not exceed 37.5°C (99.5°F).

D. The donor's oral temperature must not exceed 37.5°C (99.5°F).

44.

A. For the brief physical examination required to determine whether a blood donor is in good health, the donor's systolic blood pressure should measure 90 to 180 mm Hg. People with systolic blood pressures out of this range should be deferred as donors.

B. For the brief physical examination required to determine whether a blood donor is in good health, the donor's systolic blood pressure should measure 90 to 180 mm Hg. People with systolic blood pressures out of this range should be deferred as donors.

C. For the brief physical examination required to determine whether a blood donor is in good health, the donor's systolic blood pressure should measure 90 to 180 mm Hg. People with systolic blood pressures out of this range should be deferred as donors. (p. 353)

D. For the brief physical examination required to determine whether a blood donor is in good health, the donor's systolic blood pressure should measure 90 to 180 mm Hg. People with systolic blood pressures out of this range should be deferred as donors.

45.

A. A false-negative blood culture is more likely to occur if iodine is not wiped from the tops of the blood culture tubes, since iodine may be transferred into the blood culture tube with the needle insertion, causing inhibition of bacterial growth. (p. 335)

B. Usually, indwelling catheters are *not* used for blood culture collections, owing to the possibility of false-positive results that occur from bacterial growth occurring around the catheter.

C. Too much blood collected into the blood culture tube will more likely lead to a false-positive result.

D. If the health care worker palpates the venipuncture site after the site has been prepared without first cleaning the gloved finger, he or she can cause bacterial contamination to the blood collection site, which may lead to a false-positive result.

46.

A. The Allen test is used to compress the patient's ulnar and radial arteries to make certain that these arteries are providing collateral circulation.

B. Blood gas analysis measures pH, pO_2, and pCO_2 but not glucose.

C. To determine whether a patient suffers from lactose intolerance, a physician may order a lactose tolerance test, which involves measuring glucose levels over a 3-hour period. (pp. 344–345)

D. Therapeutic phlebotomy is the intentional removal of blood for therapeutic reasons.

47.

A. The potential blood donor will not be deferred if he or she only weighs 110 pounds.

B. A donor's oral temperature must not exceed 37.5°C. Therefore this donor's temperature was fine at 37°C.

C. The hematocrit value must be no less than 38% for blood donors. (p. 353)

D. The blood donor's pulse rate should be between 50 and 100 beats per minute.

48.

A. The presence of mild skin disorders, such as psoriasis, acne, or a poison ivy rash, does not prohibit an individual from donating unless the lesions are in the antecubital area.

B. Donors with purulent skin lesions, wounds, or severe skin infections should be deferred. The presence of mild skin disorders, such as psoriasis, acne, or a poison ivy rash, does not prohibit an individual from donating unless the lesions are in the antecubital area. (p. 353)

C. The presence of mild skin disorders, such as psoriasis, acne, or a poison ivy rash, does not prohibit an individual from donating unless the lesions are in the antecubital area.

D. The presence of mild skin disorders, such as psoriasis, acne, or a poison ivy rash, does not prohibit an individual from donating unless the lesions are in the antecubital area.

49.

A. If the blood donor is allergic to iodine, use acetone alcohol to clean the arm.

B. If the blood donor is allergic to iodine, use acetone alcohol to clean the arm.

C. If the blood donor is allergic to iodine, use acetone alcohol to clean the arm. (p. 357)

D. If the blood donor is allergic to iodine, use acetone alcohol to clean the arm.

50.

A. A fistula is an artificial shunt in which the vein and artery have been fused through surgery and is a permanent connection tube located in the arm of patients undergoing kidney dialysis.

B. A fistula is an artificial shunt in which the vein and artery have been fused through surgery and is a permanent connection tube located in the arm of patients undergoing kidney dialysis. (p. 351)

C. A fistula is an artificial shunt in which the vein and artery have been fused through surgery and is a permanent connection tube located in the arm of patients undergoing kidney dialysis.

D. A fistula is an artificial shunt in which the vein and artery have been fused through surgery and is a permanent connection tube located in the arm of patients undergoing kidney dialysis.

51.

A. Blood culture collections require special microbiology vials or SPS tubes. The special acid-washed plastic syringes would kill the microorganisms in blood culture specimens.

B. Arterial blood gas collections require arterial blood collected with heparin.

C. Glucose determinations can occur from the use of plasma, whole blood, or serum but *not* in special acid-washed plastic syringes.

D. Testing for trace metals involves the use of specially prepared trace metal evacuated blood collection tubes or special acid-washed plastic syringes. (p. 346)

52.

A. The Isostat System (Wampole Laboratories, Cranbury, NJ) is a special blood culture tube system.

B. The Simplate R (Organon Teknika Corp., Durham, NC) is a disposable device that is used to make uniform incisions for the bleeding-time test. (p. 333)

C. The BACTEC PLUS (Becton-Dickinson Diagnostic Instrument Systems, Sparks, MD) is used for blood culture collections.

D. The Allen test is a preliminary test to determine whether it is safe to collect blood from the radial artery.

53.

A. By using a butterfly assembly and transferring the blood via a direct draw adapter that fits directly over the blood culture vial (Figure 12.2), blood is transferred to the aerobic vial first since the assembly tubing contains air. (p. 337)

B. By using a butterfly assembly and transferring the blood via a direct draw adapter that fits directly over the blood culture vial (Figure 12.2), blood is transferred to the aerobic vial first since the assembly tubing contains air.

C. By using a butterfly assembly and transferring the blood via a direct draw adapter that fits directly over the blood culture vial (Figure 12.2), blood is transferred to the aerobic vial first since the assembly tubing contains air.

D. By using a butterfly assembly and transferring the blood via a direct draw adapter that fits directly over the blood culture vial (Figure 12.2), blood is transferred to the aerobic vial first since the assembly tubing contains air.

54.

A. The GTT results will be falsely affected because the test is based on a person having a carbohydrate intake that must be at least 150 grams per day for 3 days before the GTT.

B. The GTT results will be falsely affected because the test is based on a person having a carbohydrate intake that must be at least 150 grams per day for 3 days before the GTT.

C. The GTT results will be falsely affected because the test is based on a person having a carbohydrate intake that must be at least 150 grams per day for 3 days before the GTT.

D. The GTT results will be falsely affected because the test is based on a person having a carbohydrate intake that must be at least 150 grams per day for 3 days before the GTT. (p. 342)

55.

A. The purpose of the GTT is to test the patient's insulin-releasing mechanism and glucose-disposing system. (p. 342)

B. The purpose of the GTT is to test the patient's insulin-releasing mechanism and glucose-disposing system.

C. The purpose of the GTT is to test the patient's insulin-releasing mechanism and glucose-disposing system.

D. The purpose of the GTT is to test the patient's insulin-releasing mechanism and glucose-disposing system.

56.

A. For any of the blood culture collection procedures, the venipuncture site *must not* be repalpated after the venipuncture site is prepared for blood collection unless the health care worker is wearing sterile gloves and has not contaminated the finger used for palpating or the gloved finger has been cleaned with povidone-iodine before palpating the site.

B. For any of the blood culture collection procedures, the venipuncture site *must not* be repalpated after the venipuncture site is prepared for blood collection unless the health care worker is wearing sterile gloves and has not contaminated the finger used for palpating or the gloved finger has been cleaned with povidone-iodine before palpating the site.

C. For any of the blood culture collection procedures, the venipuncture site *must not* be repalpated after the venipuncture site is prepared for blood collection unless the health care worker is wearing sterile gloves and has not contaminated the finger used for palpating or the gloved finger has been cleaned with povidone-iodine before palpating the site.

D. For any of the blood culture collection procedures, the venipuncture site *must not* be repalpated after the venipuncture site is prepared for blood collection unless the health care worker is wearing sterile gloves and has not contaminated the finger used for palpating or the gloved finger has been cleaned with povidone-iodine before palpating the site. (p. 338)

57.

A. As for other usual venipuncture collections, 22- or 20-gauge is the most appropriate needle size for blood culture collections.

B. As for other usual venipuncture collections, 22- or 20-gauge is the most appropriate needle size for blood culture collections.

C. As for other usual venipuncture collections, 22- or 20-gauge is the most appropriate needle size for blood culture collections.

D. As for other usual venipuncture collections, 22- or 20-gauge is the most appropriate needle size for blood culture collections. (p. 334)

58.

A. Blood cultures are often collected from patients who have fever of unknown origin (FUO). (p. 334)

B. Blood cultures are often collected from patients who have fever of unknown origin (FUO).

C. Blood cultures are often collected from patients who have fever of unknown origin (FUO).

D. Von Willebrand's disease is a coagulation disorder that is detected through coagulation tests such as the bleeding-time test.

59.

A. One percent lidocaine is used in the arterial blood gas collection procedure to numb the site before collection.

B. One percent lidocaine is used in the arterial blood gas collection procedure to numb the site before collection. (pp. 329–330)

C. One percent lidocaine is used in the arterial blood gas collection procedure to numb the site before collection.

D. One percent lidocaine is used in the arterial blood gas collection procedure to numb the site before collection.

60.

A. Therapeutic drug-monitoring collections require the usual venipuncture blood collections with alcohol cleansing before the collection procedure. (p. 345)

B. Arterial blood gas collections require cleansing the site with povidone-iodine before collection.

C. Povidone-iodine cleansing is required for blood culture venipuncture site preparation.

D. For blood donations, the venipuncture site must be thoroughly cleansed with povidone-iodine before collection.

CHAPTER

13 Elderly, Home, and Long-term Care Collections

chapter objectives

Upon completion of Chapter 13, the learner is responsible for the following:

➤ List two terms that are synonymous with "point-of-care testing."

➤ Define five physical and/or emotional changes that are associated with the aging process.

➤ Describe how a health care worker should react to physical and emotional changes associated with the elderly.

➤ Identify four analytes whose levels can be determined through point-of-care testing.

➤ Describe the most widely used application of point-of-care testing.

➤ Given the abnormal and normal control values for glucose from a daily run, plot the control values on the appropriate quality control charts.

DIRECTIONS Each of the questions or incomplete statements below is followed by four suggested answers or completions. Select **one answer** that is best in each case.

KNOWLEDGE LEVEL = 1

1. Which of the following terms is/are synonymous with "POC testing"?
   A. alternate-site testing
   B. near-patient testing
   C. patient-focused testing
   D. all of the above

KNOWLEDGE LEVEL = 1

2. In point-of-care testing, which of the following conditions can cause erroneous results in glucose testing?
   A. waiting before specimen collection
   B. outdated reagents
   C. calibrators are not used
   D. all of the above

KNOWLEDGE LEVEL = 1

3. Trends in the elderly population indicate that point-of-service testing will increase in:
   A. day care centers
   B. homes and rehabilitation centers
   C. commercial pharmacies and health food stores
   D. Internet health sites

KNOWLEDGE LEVEL = 1

4. Hearing loss is common among the elderly and may cause embarrassment or frustration. Which of the following accommodations would be most appropriate and can easily be made to facilitate the specimen collection process?

   A. speak very loudly and forcefully
   B. adjust one's position to speak into the "good" ear
   C. give the patient printed instructions so that verbal communication is not necessary
   D. use a microphone

KNOWLEDGE LEVEL = 1

5. Physical frailties that may affect elderly individuals include:
   A. loss of taste, smell, and feeling
   B. memory loss about taking medications
   C. susceptibility to hypothermia
   D. all of the above

KNOWLEDGE LEVEL = 1

6. Which of the following abbreviations refer(s) to the term "hematocrit"?
   A. Hct, crit
   B. CBC
   C. hemo scan
   D. none of the above

KNOWLEDGE LEVEL = 1

7. Which of the following blood assays can assist in the diagnosis and evaluation of anemia?
   A. Na^+, K^+
   B. hemoglobin and hematocrit
   C. glucose and insulin
   D. all of the above

KNOWLEDGE LEVEL = 1

8. In terms of quality control procedures, "SD" stands for:

   A. short distance

   B. standand deviation

   C. shared diameter

   D. standard dimension

For Questions 9–12, please refer to Figure 13.1 if necessary.

 KNOWLEDGE LEVEL = 2

9. Interpretation of a quality control chart is based on the fact that for a normal distribution:

   A. 99% of the values are within 3 SD of the mean

   B. 99% of the values are within 2 SD of the mean

   C. 95% of the values are within 3 SD of the mean

   D. 95% of the values are within 1 SD of the mean

 KNOWLEDGE LEVEL = 2

10. Using Figure 13.1, which of the following statements is true?

   A. On day 7, the glucose control was out of the 2 SD control range.

   B. On day 8, the glucose control was the same as the patient's value.

   C. On day 3, the glucose control had a mean value of 100 mg/dL.

   D. On day 1 the glucose control was too low.

 KNOWLEDGE LEVEL = 2

11. Using Figure 13.1, identify the tolerance limits for the glucose control.

   A. 91 to 100 mg/dL

   B. 100 to 109 mg/dL

   C. 91 to 109 mg/dL

   D. 96 to 105 mg/dL

 KNOWLEDGE LEVEL = 2

12. When referring to a quality control chart like Figure 13.1, what do the comments indicate?

   A. There was a problem on day 2 and day 5.

   B. There was a dead battery on day 5.

   C. Preventative maintenance was properly documented.

   D. all of the above

 KNOWLEDGE LEVEL = 1

13. Which of the following is released from the pancreas and has a major effect on blood glucose levels?

   A. ACTH

   B. insulin

   C. thyroxine

   D. renin

 KNOWLEDGE LEVEL = 1

14. Most rapid methods for glucose testing require:

   A. serum

   B. plasma

   C. skin puncture blood

   D. red blood cells

 KNOWLEDGE LEVEL = 1

15. Na^+, K^+, Cl^-, and HCO^- are usually referred to as:

   A. electrolytes

   B. blood gases

   C. hormones

   D. coagulation factors

FIGURE 13.1. Quality control record.

QUALITY CONTROL RECORD

PRACTICE NAME

PRECISION HEALTH CARE INC.

INSTRUMENT *Glucose Monitor- Institution #55*

NAME/LEVEL

CONTROL LOT # *11542A*　　　EXPIRATION DATE *01/29/99*

Director Signature/Date:

TEST *Glucose*　*Glucose Monitor*　　UNITS *mg/dl*

LOWER LIMIT *91*　　MEAN *100*　　UPPER LIMIT *109*

DATE	No.	VALUE	TECH	COMMENT	DATE	No.	VALUE	TECH	COMMENT
12/8/98	1	99				17			
12/9/98	2	103		prev. maintenance		18			
12/10/98	3	100				19			
12/11/98	4	100				20			
12/14/98	5	105				21			
12/15/98	6	97				22			
12/16/98	7	95				23			
12/17/98	8	96		new battery		24			
12/18/98	9	103				25			
12/19/98	10	100				26			
12/20/98	11	103				27			
12/21/98	12	97				28			
	13					29			
	14					30			
	15					31			
	16								

DATE:

109 UPPER LIMIT

100 MEAN

91 LOWER LIMIT

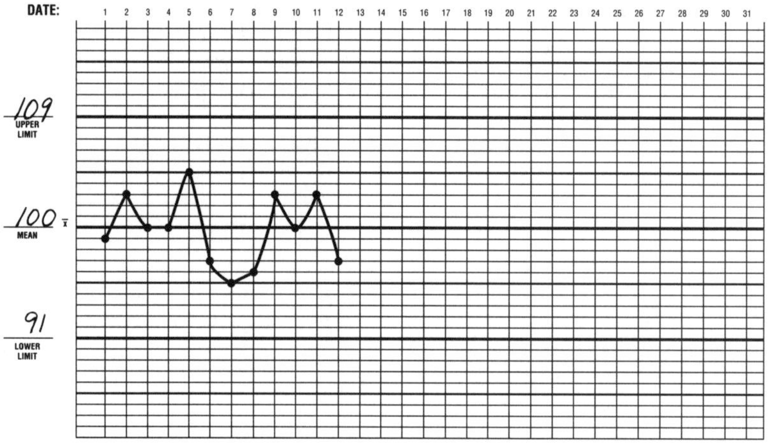

 KNOWLEDGE LEVEL = 1

16. What is troponin T?
    A. a coagulation factor
    B. an instrument that is used to test T_4
    C. protein that is released after a myocardial infarction
    D. an electrolyte

 KNOWLEDGE LEVEL = 2

17. What should a health care worker do before using reagent strips and/or controls in point-of-care testing?
    A. Check the date that the bottle was opened.
    B. Check the expiration date.
    C. Ensure proper storage temperature.
    D. all of the above

KNOWLEDGE LEVEL = 1

18. Specimen collection in a patient's home may involve unusual positioning of the patient. What is the preferred position or location from which to collect a blood specimen from a homebound patient?
    A. in the bathroom
    B. in a comfortable, reclining position
    C. seated next to the kitchen table
    D. all of the above

 KNOWLEDGE LEVEL = 1

19. Transportation requirements for specimens collected from homebound patients include:
    A. leakproof containers
    B. cooling or heating accommodations
    C. timing efficiency in returning to the laboratory
    D. all of the above

 KNOWLEDGE LEVEL = 1

20. Extra supplies and equipment are needed by home health care workers who collect specimens from homebound patients that are *not* necessary for workers in a hospital. These include:
    A. map and wireless phone
    B. biohazard container
    C. hand disinfectant
    D. all of the above

 KNOWLEDGE LEVEL = 1

21. Which of the following is an acceptable alternative to hand washing?
    A. cream or foam disinfectants
    B. wearing gloves
    C. diluted chlorox spray
    D. none of the above

 KNOWLEDGE LEVEL = 1

22. Which of the following is a debilitating disease causing tremors, particularly in elderly individuals?
    A. anemia
    B. Parkinson's disease
    C. Alzheimer's disease
    D. all of the above

 KNOWLEDGE LEVEL = 1

23. Emotional factors that are associated with the aging process include:
    A. loss of career or retirement
    B. loss of spouse
    C. depression
    D. all of the above

 KNOWLEDGE LEVEL = 1

24. Results from point-of-care testing should contain:
    A. the exact same information as results from a clinical laboratory
    B. the same information as results from a clinical laboratory and a note that the results are from a bedside (or home) rather than the clinical lab
    C. a signature from the patient
    D. an informed consent from the patient

 KNOWLEDGE LEVEL = 1

25. Most instruments manufactured for glucose testing have which of the following features?
    A. reagent strip or pad
    B. reader to record a color reaction
    C. buzzer or alarm to alert the health care worker
    D. all of the above

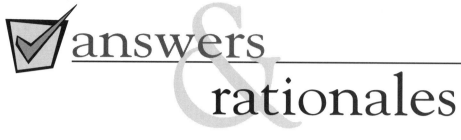

1.

A. The demand for point-of-care (POC) testing is increasing because rapid turnaround of laboratory results is necessary for prompt medical decision making. This type of testing occurs at or near the point of direct contact with the patient. Therefore the terms used for these direct laboratory services include decentralized lab testing, on-site testing, alternate-site testing, near-patient testing, patient-focused testing, and bedside testing.

B. The demand for point-of-care (POC) testing is increasing because rapid turnaround of laboratory results is necessary for prompt medical decision making. This type of testing occurs at or near the point of direct contact with the patient. Therefore the terms used for these direct laboratory services include decentralized lab testing, on-site testing, alternate-site testing, near-patient testing, patient-focused testing, and bedside testing.

C. The demand for point-of-care (POC) testing is increasing because rapid turnaround of laboratory results is necessary for prompt medical decision making. This type of testing occurs at or near the point of direct contact with the patient. Therefore the terms used for these direct laboratory services include decentralized lab testing, on-site testing, alternate-site testing, near-patient testing, patient-focused testing, and bedside testing.

D. The demand for point-of-care (POC) testing is increasing because rapid turnaround of laboratory results is necessary for prompt medical decision making. This type of testing occurs at or near the point of direct contact with the patient. Therefore the terms used for these direct laboratory services include decentralized lab testing, on-site testing, alternate-site testing, near-patient testing, patient-focused testing, and bedside testing. (p. 368)

2.

A. There are many conditions to be careful about and avoid when performing point-of-care glucose testing. These include improper storage of the specimen, contamination of the blood with alcohol, collection of the specimen at the wrong time or after excessive waiting, techniques that are not performed to the manufacturer's recommendations, unclean instruments, outdated or improperly stored reagents, improperly used calibrators and/or controls, and identification or labeling errors.

B. There are many conditions to be careful about and avoid when performing point-of-care glucose testing. These include improper storage of the specimen, contamination of the blood with alcohol, collection of the specimen at the wrong time or after excessive waiting, techniques that are not performed to the manufacturer's recommendations, unclean instruments, outdated or improperly stored reagents, improperly used calibrators and/or controls, and identification or labeling errors.

C. There are many conditions to be careful about and avoid when performing point-of-care glucose testing. These include improper storage of the specimen, contamination of the blood with alcohol, collection of the specimen at the wrong time or after excessive waiting, techniques that are not performed to the manufacturer's recommendations, unclean instruments, outdated or improperly stored reagents, improperly used calibrators and/or controls, and identification or labeling errors.

D. There are many conditions to be careful about and avoid when performing point-of-care glucose testing. These include improper storage of the specimen, contamination of the blood with alcohol, collection of the specimen at the wrong time or after excessive waiting, techniques that are not performed to the manufacturer's recommendations, unclean instruments, outdated or improperly stored reagents, improperly used calibrators and/or controls, and identification or labeling errors. (p. 374)

3.

A. Day care centers are less likely to provide health services involving laboratory testing.

B. Trends in the elderly population indicate that point-of-service testing will increase in patients' homes (home health care), nursing homes (skilled nursing facilities), rehabilitation centers, and other types of long-term care facilities. (p. 368)

C. Commercial pharmacies and health food stores are less likely to offer health services involving laboratory testing.

D. Internet health sites cannot realistically conduct point-of-care testing; however, there are sites that offer advice and/or products that can be used for point-of-care testing.

4.

A. Speaking very loudly and forcefully is not necessary and can be perceived as disrespectful and rude behavior.

B. Hearing loss is common among the elderly. However, not all elderly people are affected by it, and the severity of the problem varies widely. Elderly individuals should be treated with the utmost respect and dignity. Simply repeating the instructions or adjusting one's position to speak into the "good" ear may be all that is needed to ensure the patient's understanding. (p. 368)

C. Giving the patient printed instructions may be a good idea, especially if the degree of deafness is significant, but written instructions should not take the place of a professional, informative dialog. Verbal communication is also necessary because it provides reassurance to the patient and enables the health care worker to check for understanding.

D. Use of a microphone would likely be distracting, embarrassing, and humiliating to the patient.

5.

A. Physical frailties that may affect elderly individuals include loss of taste, smell, and feeling; memory loss about taking medications; susceptibility to hypothermia; and muscular degeneration.

B. Physical frailties that may affect elderly individuals include loss of taste, smell, and feeling; memory loss about taking medications; susceptibility to hypothermia; and muscular degeneration.

C. Physical frailties that may affect elderly individuals include loss of taste, smell, and feeling; memory loss about taking medications; susceptibility to hypothermia; and muscular degeneration.

D. Physical frailties that may affect elderly individuals include loss of taste, smell, and feeling; memory loss about taking medications; susceptibility to hypothermia; and muscular degeneration. (p. 368)

6.

A. The abbreviations "Hct" and "crit" are synonymous with the term "hematocrit." (p. 379)

B. "CBC" is the abbreviation for "complete blood count."

C. "Hemo scan" is not a term that is used for a hematocrit test.

D. "None of the above" is incorrect.

7.

A. Sodium and potassium determinations (Na$^+$, K$^+$) are important laboratory tests to evaluate electrolyte balance.

B. Laboratory evaluations of hemoglobin and hematocrit assist in the diagnosis and evaluation of anemia. (p. 379)

C. Glucose and insulin determinations are useful in diagnosing, monitoring, and treating diabetes.

D. "All of the above" is incorrect.

8.

A. "Short distance" is not a quality control term.

B. "SD" stands for "standard deviation." It is used in quality control procedures to determine variation from the mean, or the average value that is expected. In a normal distribution of values, 95% of the time the values will be within 2 standard deviations of the mean, and 99% of the values are within 3 standard deviations of the mean. (p. 372)

C. "Shared diameter" is not a quality control term.

D. "Standard dimension" is not a quality control term.

9.

A. Interpretation of a quality control chart is based on the fact that for a normal distribution, 99% of the values are within 3 SD of the mean. (p. 372)

B. In a normal distribution, 99% of the values are not within 2 SD of the mean; only 95% of the values are within 2 SD.

C. In a normal distribution, 99%, not 95%, of the values are within 3 SD of the mean.

D. In a normal distribution, 95% of the values are within 2 SD, not 1 SD of the mean.

10.

A. On day 7, the glucose control was *not* out of the 2 SD control range.

B. This quality control chart is not an evaluation of the patient's glucose level. It only reflects measurements of the glucose control (lot # 11542A that expired on 01/29/99).

C. On day 3, the glucose control had a value of 100 mg/dL, which happens to be the mean value. This is normal and expected. (p. 372)

D. On day 1, the glucose control was *not* too low; it was within 1 SD of the mean.

11.

A. The range 91-100 mg/dL reflects only values within 2 standard deviations *below* the mean.

B. The range 100-109 mg/dL reflects only values within 2 standard deviations *above* the mean.

C. The tolerance limits for the glucose control are from 91 mg/dL (lower limit) to 109 mg/dL (upper limit). (p. 372)

D. This range (96-105 mg/dL) is *within* the tolerance limits of the quality control chart.

12.

A. There was not a problem on day 2 or day 5.

B. There probably was not a dead battery on day 5; rather, there should have been a replaced battery as scheduled by required maintenance.

C. The comments indicate that preventative maintenance was properly documented, and a battery was replaced as is probably indicated in the required maintenance of the instrument. (p. 372)

D. "All of the above" is incorrect.

13.

A. ACTH (adrenocorticotropic hormone) determinations are useful in assessing endocrine system abnormalities. It is not released from the pancreas.

B. Insulin is released from the pancreas and has a major effect on blood glucose levels. Normally, insulin is released into the bloodstream after meals when glucose levels increase; it causes glucose to be absorbed from the blood into the body tissues where it is used for energy. In patients with diabetes mellitus, glucose is not properly absorbed by the tissues, and the glucose levels within the blood increase. If a patient has an elevated level, he or she can enter a state of metabolic acidosis, which in turn may result in shock and death. (p. 369)

C. Thyroxine (T_4) determinations are used to assess thyroid function. It is not released from the pancreas.

D. Renin determinations are useful in assessing endocrine system abnormalities. It is not released from the pancreas.

14.

A. Since serum requires more time to prepare for testing, skin puncture blood is more commonly used for *rapid* procedures.

B. Plasma may also be used; however, skin puncture blood provides a more immediate sample for testing.

C. Most rapid methods for glucose testing require skin puncture blood. (p. 370)

D. Red blood cells alone are not used for rapid glucose testing.

15.

A. Na^+, K^+, Cl^-, and HCO^- are usually referred to as electrolytes. (p. 374)

B. Blood gas analyses include measurement of the partial pressure of oxygen, carbon dioxide, and blood pH.

C. Hormone levels are usually associated with evaluation of the endocrine or reproductive systems.

D. Coagulation factors evaluate bleeding and clotting potential.

16.

A. Troponin T is not a coagulation factor.

B. Troponin T is not an instrument that is used to test T_4.

C. Troponin T is a protein that is released after a myocardial infarction. (p. 376)

D. Troponin T is not an electrolyte.

17.

A. Point-of-care testing requires careful attention to quality control measures and details. Before using reagent strips and/or controls in point-of-care testing, a health care worker should check the date that the bottle was opened, check the expiration date, and ensure proper storage temperature.

B. Point-of-care testing requires careful attention to quality control measures and details. Before using reagent strips and/or controls in point-of-care testing, a health care worker should check the date that the bottle was opened, check the expiration date, and ensure proper storage temperature.

C. Point-of-care testing requires careful attention to quality control measures and details. Before using reagent strips and/or controls in point-of-care testing, a health care worker should check the date that the bottle was opened, check the expiration date, and ensure proper storage temperature.

D. Point-of-care testing requires careful attention to quality control measures and details. Before using reagent strips and/or controls in point-of-care testing, a health care worker should check the date that the bottle was opened, check the expiration date, and ensure proper storage temperature. (pp. 370–374)

18.

A. In performing specimen collection procedures in the home, it is important for the health care worker to identify where the bathroom is in relation to the patient. This way, the health care worker can easily wash hands or perhaps even use clean towels if available.

B. The preferred position/location from which to collect a blood specimen from a homebound patient is in a comfortable, reclining position so that the patient does not fall if he or she faints. (p. 369)

C. The preferred position is in a reclining one for safety sake. When a patient is seated next to the kitchen table, there is a greater possibility of injury if he or she falls out of a chair after fainting. Often, there is no one else who can assist the health care worker if this scenario occurs.

D. "All of the above" is incorrect.

19.

A. Transportation requirements for specimens collected from homebound patients include use of leakproof containers, ensuring appropriate temperature requirements by using cooling or heating instruments, and careful attention to timing when returning specimens to the laboratory for testing. Delays should be well documented.

B. Transportation requirements for specimens collected from homebound patients include use of leakproof containers, ensuring appropriate temperature requirements by using cooling or heating instruments, and careful attention to timing when returning specimens to the laboratory for testing. Delays should be well documented.

C. Transportation requirements for specimens collected from homebound patients include use of leakproof containers, ensuring appropriate temperature requirements by using cooling or heating instruments, and careful attention to timing when returning specimens to the laboratory for testing. Delays should be well documented.

D. Transportation requirements for specimens collected from homebound patients include use of leakproof containers, ensuring appropriate temperature requirements by using cooling or heating instruments, and careful attention to timing when returning specimens to the laboratory for testing. Delays should be well documented. (p. 369)

20.

A. Extra supplies and equipment needed by home health care workers who collect specimens from homebound patients that are *not* necessary for workers in a hospital are a map and a wireless phone. The map prevents the worker from getting lost en route to or from the home. The phone is helpful under difficult or emergency circumstances. (p. 369)

B. A biohazard container is necessary both for workers in a hospital and in the home.

C. Hand disinfectant or hand washing is necessary for workers both in a hospital and in the home.

D. "All of the above" is incorrect.

21.

A. Using cream or foam disinfectants is an acceptable alternative to hand washing. This may be particularly helpful in the home setting if conditions are not very clean. (p. 369)

B. Wearing gloves should always occur and is not a substitute for hand washing.

C. Using diluted chlorox spray on one's hands is not a good substitute for hand washing.

D. "None of the above" is incorrect.

22.

A. Anemia is not necessarily associated with the aging process and does not cause tremors.

B. Parkinson's disease is a debilitating disease causing tremors, particularly in elderly individuals. (p. 368)

C. Alzheimer's disease is also associated with the aging process; however, it affects the mind.

D. "All of the above" is incorrect.

23.

A. Emotional factors that are associated with the aging process include loss of career or retirement, loss of spouse or close friends, and depression or anger at life.

B. Emotional factors that are associated with the aging process include loss of career or retirement, loss of spouse or close friends, and depression or anger at life.

C. Emotional factors that are associated with the aging process include loss of career or retirement, loss of spouse or close friends, and depression or anger at life.

D. Emotional factors that are associated with the aging process include loss of career or retirement, loss of spouse or close friends, and depression or anger at life. (pp. 368–369)

24.

A. Results should contain the exact same information as results from a clinical laboratory in addition to a note about the site of testing (bedside or home testing).

B. Results from point-of-care testing should contain the same information as results from a clinical laboratory plus a note that the results are from a bedside (or home) rather than the clinical laboratory. (p. 371)

C. A signature from the patient is not necessary on the test results.

D. An informed consent from the patient is needed but not on the results of the laboratory test.

25.

A. Most instruments manufactured for POC glucose testing have a reagent strip or pad, a reader to record a color reaction on the strip/pad, and a buzzer or alarm to alert the health care worker that it is time to read the result. Timing of the reaction is critical.

B. Most instruments manufactured for POC glucose testing have a reagent strip or pad, a reader to record a color reaction on the strip/pad, and a buzzer or alarm to alert the health care worker that it is time to read the result. Timing of the reaction is critical.

C. Most instruments manufactured for POC glucose testing have a reagent strip or pad, a reader to record a color reaction on the strip/pad, and a buzzer or alarm to alert the health care worker that it is time to read the result. Timing of the reaction is critical.

D. Most instruments manufactured for POC glucose testing have a reagent strip or pad, a reader to record a color reaction on the strip/pad, and a buzzer or alarm to alert the health care worker that it is time to read the result. Timing of the reaction is critical. (p. 371)

14 Urinalysis and Body Fluid Collections

chapter objectives

Upon completion of Chapter 14, the learner is responsible for the following:

➤ Identify the types of body fluid specimens, other than blood, that are analyzed in the clinical laboratory and the correct procedures for collecting and/or transporting these specimens to the laboratory.

➤ Identify the various types of specimens collected for microbiological, throat, and nasopharyngeal cultures and the protocol that health care workers must follow when transporting these specimens.

➤ List the types of patient specimens that are needed for gastric and sweat chloride analyses.

➤ List three types of urine specimen collections and differentiate the uses of the urine specimens obtained from these collections.

DIRECTIONS Each of the questions or incomplete statements below is followed by four suggested answers or completions. Select **one answer** that is best in each case.

 KNOWLEDGE LEVEL = 3

1. The first analyte that can be detected in urine or serum produced in pregnancy is:
   A. PRL
   B. HCG
   C. ACTH
   D. TSH

 KNOWLEDGE LEVEL = 1

2. For the urinary pregnancy test, the preferred urine specimen is a:
   A. 2-hour urine collection
   B. 24-hour urine sample
   C. random urine sample
   D. clean-catch midstream sample

 KNOWLEDGE LEVEL = 2

3. Which of the following is obtained through a lumbar puncture?
   A. pleural fluid
   B. cerebrospinal fluid
   C. synovial fluid
   D. peritoneal fluid

 KNOWLEDGE LEVEL = 2

4. Nasopharyngeal culture collections may be used to diagnose:
   A. whooping cough
   B. *Salmonella* infection
   C. *Shigella* infection
   D. *Crytococcus* infection

 KNOWLEDGE LEVEL = 1

5. Fluid composed of products formed in various male reproductive organs is referred to as:
   A. pleural fluid
   B. seminal fluid
   C. synovial fluid
   D. cerebrospinal fluid

 KNOWLEDGE LEVEL = 1

6. The Hollander test is run on
   A. synovial fluid
   B. gastric secretions
   C. urine
   D. CSF

 KNOWLEDGE LEVEL = 2

7. Which of the following types of urine specimens is the "cleanest," or least contaminated?
   A. first morning specimen
   B. timed specimen
   C. midstream specimen
   D. random specimen

 KNOWLEDGE LEVEL = 1

8. Creatinine clearance is determined through use of:
   A. urine specimens
   B. pericardial fluid specimens
   C. synovial fluid
   D. CSF specimens

KNOWLEDGE LEVEL = 1

9. Amniotic fluid can be found:
   A. around the lungs
   B. surrounding the heart
   C. around the fetus in the uterus
   D. surrounding the liver, the pancreas, and other parts of the gastrointestinal area

 KNOWLEDGE LEVEL = 1

10. A urine C & S should be performed on a:
   A. random urine sample
   B. clean-catch midstream sample
   C. routine urine sample
   D. 24-hour urine specimen

 KNOWLEDGE LEVEL = 1

11. Peritoneal fluid is located:
   A. around the lungs
   B. in the joints
   C. in the abdomen
   D. in the sac around the heart

 KNOWLEDGE LEVEL = 2

12. A 24-hour urine specimen is usually collected to test for:
   A. hormones
   B. glucose
   C. creatine kinase
   D. bacteria

 KNOWLEDGE LEVEL = 1

13. Pericardial fluid is collected from the
   A. abdomen
   B. sac around the heart
   C. joints
   D. sac around the lungs

 KNOWLEDGE LEVEL = 2

14. Skin tests are used to determine whether a patient has ever had contact with:
   A. a particular antibody and has produced antigens to that antibody
   B. a particular antigen and has produced antibodies to that antigen
   C. the disease leukemia
   D. the disease polycythemia

 KNOWLEDGE LEVEL = 1

15. The fluid collected from a joint cavity is:
   A. peritoneal fluid
   B. pleural fluid
   C. abdominal fluid
   D. synovial fluid

 KNOWLEDGE LEVEL = 2

16. Throat cultures are most commonly obtained to determine the presence of:
   A. *Neisseria* infection
   B. *Streptococcus* infection
   C. *Staphylococcus* infection
   D. *Bacillus* infection

 KNOWLEDGE LEVEL = 1

17. The best site for a sweat chloride test on a child is the:
   A. arm
   B. hand
   C. leg
   D. finger

KNOWLEDGE LEVEL = 2

18. What type of urine specimen is needed to detect an infection?
    A. random
    B. clean-catch
    C. routine
    D. 24-hour

 KNOWLEDGE LEVEL = 1

19. Which of the following types of specimens is most frequently collected for analysis?
    A. amniotic fluid
    B. urine
    C. CSF
    D. pericardial fluid

 KNOWLEDGE LEVEL = 1

20. The O & P analysis is requested on:
    A. CSF specimens
    B. amniotic fluid specimens
    C. fecal specimens
    D. synovial fluid specimens

 KNOWLEDGE LEVEL = 1

21. The occult blood analysis is frequently requested on:
    A. CSF specimens
    B. fecal specimens
    C. throat cultures
    D. seminal fluid specimens

 KNOWLEDGE LEVEL = 2

22. Ketosis is frequently associated with:
    A. liver disease
    B. diabetes mellitus
    C. chemical poisoning
    D. infection

 KNOWLEDGE LEVEL = 2

23. Which of the following can be used in children and infants to diagnose whooping cough?
    A. Hollander test
    B. nasopharyngeal culture
    C. O & P test
    D. sweat chloride test

 KNOWLEDGE LEVEL = 1

24. The sweat chloride test is used to diagnose:
    A. cerebral palsy
    B. multiple sclerosis
    C. cystic fibrosis
    D. diabetes mellitus

 KNOWLEDGE LEVEL = 1

25. What is the specimen of choice for drug abuse testing?
    A. CSF
    B. gastric fluid
    C. synovial fluid
    D. urine

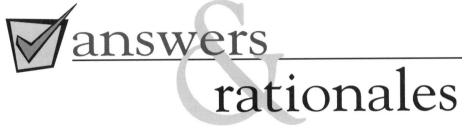

answers & rationales

1.

A. Prolactin (PRL) is a hormone produced in the female but is not the first analyte detected in urine or serum in pregnancy.

B. Human chorionic gonadotropin (HCG) is the first detectable analyte produced in pregnancy. (p. 389)

C. Adrenocorticotropic hormone (ACTH) is a hormone produced in the pituitary gland and is *not* the first analyte detected in urine or serum in pregnancy.

D. Thyroid-stimulating hormone (TSH) is associated with thyroid activities, and thus, is not used as an analyte to detect pregnancy.

2.

A. A random urine sample is the specimen of choice for a urinary pregnancy test.

B. A random urine sample is the specimen of choice for a urinary pregnancy test.

C. A random urine sample is the specimen of choice for a urinary pregnancy test. (p. 389)

D. A random urine sample is the specimen of choice for a urinary pregnancy test.

3.

A. Pleural fluid is obtained from the lung cavity.

B. Cerebrospinal fluid (CSF) is obtained by a physician through a spinal tap or lumbar puncture. (p. 394)

C. Synovial fluid is obtained aseptically from joint cavities.

D. Peritoneal fluid is obtained from the abdominal cavity.

4.

A. Nasopharyngeal culture collections may be used to diagnose whooping cough. (p. 396)

B. Nasopharyngeal culture collections may be used to diagnose whooping cough.

C. Nasopharyngeal culture collections may be used to diagnose whooping cough.

D. Nasopharyngeal culture collections may be used to diagnose whooping cough.

5.

A. Pleural fluid is in the lungs.

B. Seminal fluid is composed of products formed in various male reproductive organs. (p. 395)

C. Synovial fluid is in the joints.

D. Cerebrospinal fluid is in the spinal column and contains numerous analytes, including protein, glucose, and chloride.

6.

A. The Hollander test determines gastric function in terms of stomach acid production and is run on gastric secretions.

B. The Hollander test determines gastric function in terms of stomach acid production and is run on gastric secretions. (p. 397)

C. The Hollander test determines gastric function in terms of stomach acid production and is run on gastric secretions.

D. The Hollander test determines gastric function in terms of stomach acid production and is run on gastric secretions.

7.

A. The midstream, or clean-catch, specimen is the "cleanest" or least-contaminated urine specimen.

B. The midstream, or clean-catch, specimen is the "cleanest" or least-contaminated urine specimen.

C. The midstream, or clean-catch, specimen is the "cleanest" or least-contaminated urine specimen. (pp. 390–391)

D. The midstream, or clean-catch, specimen is the "cleanest" or least-contaminated urine specimen.

8.

A. The creatinine clearance used to determine kidney damage is based on results from urine and blood specimens. (p. 392)

B. The creatinine clearance used to determine kidney damage is based on results from urine and blood specimens.

C. The creatinine clearance used to determine kidney damage is based on results from urine and blood specimens.

D. The creatinine clearance used to determine kidney damage is based on results from urine and blood specimens.

9.

A. Pleural fluid is in the lung cavity.

B. Pericardial fluid surrounds the heart.

C. Amniotic fluid surrounds the fetus in the uterus. (p. 395)

D. Peritoneal fluid is within the abdominal cavity.

10.

A. A urine culture and sensitivity (C & S) test requires a clean-catch midstream urine collection to avoid contamination.

B. A urine culture and sensitivity (C & S) test requires a clean-catch midstream urine collection to avoid contamination. (p. 390)

C. A urine culture and sensitivity (C & S) test requires a clean-catch midstream urine collection to avoid contamination.

D. A urine culture and sensitivity (C & S) test requires a clean-catch midstream urine collection to avoid contamination.

11.

A. Pleural fluid is located in the lung cavity.

B. Synovial fluid is found in the joints.

C. Peritoneal fluid is located in the abdomen. (p. 395)

D. Pericardial fluid is located in the sac around the heart.

12.

A. A 24-hour urine specimen is usually collected to test for hormone studies or the creatinine clearance. (p. 392)

B. A 24-hour urine specimen is usually collected to test for hormone studies or the creatinine clearance.

C. A 24-hour urine specimen is usually collected to test for hormone studies or the creatinine clearance.

D. A 24-hour urine specimen is usually collected to test for hormone studies or the creatinine clearance.

13.

A. Peritoneal fluid is collected from the abdominal cavity.

B. Pericardial fluid is collected from the sac around the heart. (p. 395)

C. Synovial fluid is collected from the abdominal cavity.

D. Pleural fluid is collected from the sac around the lungs.

14.

A. Skin tests are used to determine whether a patient has ever had contact with a particular antigen and has produced antibodies to that antigen.

B. Skin tests are used to determine whether a patient has ever had contact with a particular antigen and has produced antibodies to that antigen. (p. 396)

C. Skin tests are used to determine whether a patient has ever had contact with a particular antigen and has produced antibodies to that antigen.

D. Skin tests are used to determine whether a patient has ever had contact with a particular antigen and has produced antibodies to that antigen.

15.

A. Peritoneal fluid is collected from the abdominal cavity.

B. Pleural fluid is collected from the lung cavity.

C. The fluid collected from a joint cavity is synovial fluid.

D. The fluid collected from a joint cavity is synovial fluid. (p. 395)

16.

A. Throat cultures are most commonly obtained to determine the presence of a streptococcal infection.

B. Throat cultures are most commonly obtained to determine the presence of a streptococcal infection. (p. 396)

C. Throat cultures are most commonly obtained to determine the presence of a streptococcal infection.

D. Throat cultures are most commonly obtained to determine the presence of a streptococcal infection.

17.

A. To perform the sweat chloride test on a child, the health care worker should choose a site with a large surface area; the best site is the leg.

B. To perform the sweat chloride test on a child, the health care worker should choose a site with a large surface area; the best site is the leg.

C. To perform the sweat chloride test on a child, the health care worker should choose a site with a large surface area; the best site is the leg. (p. 398)

D. To perform the sweat chloride test on a child, the health care worker should choose a site with a large surface area; the best site is the leg.

18.

A. The clean-catch urine specimen is used to detect the presence or absence of infecting organisms. Therefore the specimen is collected in such a manner as to avoid contamination by bacteria on the external genital areas.

B. The clean-catch urine specimen is used to detect the presence or absence of infecting organisms. Therefore the specimen is collected in such a manner as to avoid contamination by bacteria on the external genital areas. (p. 390)

C. The clean-catch urine specimen is used to detect the presence or absence of infecting organisms. Therefore, the specimen is collected in such a manner as to avoid contamination by bacteria on the external genital areas.

D. The clean-catch urine specimen is used to detect the presence or absence of infecting organisms. Therefore, the specimen is collected in such a manner as to avoid contamination by bacteria on the external genital areas.

19.

A. Routine urinalysis is one of the most frequently requested laboratory procedures because it can provide a useful indication of body health.

B. Routine urinalysis is one of the most frequently requested laboratory procedures because it can provide a useful indication of body health. (p. 388)

C. Routine urinalysis is one of the most frequently requested laboratory procedures because it can provide a useful indication of body health.

D. Routine urinalysis is one of the most frequently requested laboratory procedures because it can provide a useful indication of body health.

20.

A. Stool (fecal) specimens are commonly collected to detect parasites, such as ova and parasites (O & P), enteric disease organisms, and viruses.

B. Stool (fecal) specimens are commonly collected to detect parasites, such as ova and parasites (O & P), enteric disease organisms, and viruses.

C. Stool (fecal) specimens are commonly collected to detect parasites, such as ova and parasites (O & P), enteric disease organisms, and viruses. (p. 394)

D. Stool (fecal) specimens are commonly collected to detect parasites, such as ova and parasites (O & P), enteric disease organisms, and viruses.

21.

A. Laboratory determination of occult (invisible) blood in feces can assist in the confirmation of the presence of blood in black stools and be helpful in detecting gastrointestinal tract lesions and colorectal cancer.

B. Laboratory determination of occult (invisible) blood in feces can assist in the confirmation of the presence of blood in black stools and be helpful in detecting gastrointestinal tract lesions and colorectal cancer. (p. 394)

C. Laboratory determination of occult (invisible) blood in feces can assist in the confirmation of the presence of blood in black stools and be helpful in detecting gastrointestinal tract lesions and colorectal cancer.

D. Laboratory determination of occult (invisible) blood in feces can assist in the confirmation of the presence of blood in black stools and be helpful in detecting gastrointestinal tract lesions and colorectal cancer.

22.

A. Ketosis (presence of ketone bodies in urine) is frequently detected in patients who have diabetes mellitus.

B. Ketosis (presence of ketone bodies in urine) is frequently detected in patients who have diabetes mellitus. (p. 388)

C. Ketosis (presence of ketone bodies in urine) is frequently detected in patients who have diabetes mellitus.

D. Ketosis (presence of ketone bodies in urine) is frequently detected in patients who have diabetes mellitus.

23.

A. A nasopharyngeal culture is often performed to detect carrier states of bacteria such as *Haemophilus influenzae* and *Staphylococcus aureus*. In children and infants, this type of culture can be used to diagnose whooping cough, croup, and pneumonia.

B. A nasopharyngeal culture is often performed to detect carrier states of bacteria such as *Haemophilus influenzae* and *Staphylococcus aureus*. In children and infants, this type of culture can be used to diagnose whooping cough, croup, and pneumonia. (p. 396)

C. A nasopharyngeal culture is often performed to detect carrier states of bacteria such as *Haemophilus influenzae* and *Staphylococcus aureus*. In children and infants, this type of culture can be used to diagnose whooping cough, croup, and pneumonia.

D. A nasopharyngeal culture is often performed to detect carrier states of bacteria such as *Haemophilus influenzae* and *Staphylococcus aureus*. In children and infants, this type of culture can be used to diagnose whooping cough, croup, and pneumonia.

24.

A. The sweat chloride test is used in the diagnosis of cystic fibrosis. Cystic fibrosis is a disorder of the exocrine glands.

B. The sweat chloride test is used in the diagnosis of cystic fibrosis. Cystic fibrosis is a disorder of the exocrine glands.

C. The sweat chloride test is used in the diagnosis of cystic fibrosis. Cystic fibrosis is a disorder of the exocrine glands. (p. 397)

D. The sweat chloride test is used in the diagnosis of cystic fibrosis. Cystic fibrosis is a disorder of the exocrine glands.

25.

A. Urine is the specimen of choice for drug abuse testing. The end product metabolites of drugs, as well as the drugs, are excreted in the urine.

B. Urine is the specimen of choice for drug abuse testing. The end product metabolites of drugs, as well as the drugs, are excreted in the urine.

C. Urine is the specimen of choice for drug abuse testing. The end product metabolites of drugs, as well as the drugs, are excreted in the urine.

D. Urine is the specimen of choice for drug abuse testing. The end product metabolites of drugs, as well as the drugs, are excreted in the urine. (p. 389)

15 Specimen Collection for Forensic Toxicology, Workplace Testing, Sports Medicine

chapter objectives

Upon completion of Chapter 15, the learner is responsible for the following:

➤ Define "toxicology" and "forensic toxicology."

➤ Give five examples of specimens that can be used for forensic analysis.

➤ Describe the role of the health care worker or "collector" in federal drug testing programs.

➤ List security measures and minimum site requirements for urine collection for federal drug testing programs.

➤ Describe the function of a chain-of-custody, and the Custody and Control form.

➤ List the basic steps in specimen collection for urine drug tests and blood alcohol levels.

DIRECTIONS Each of the questions or incomplete statements below is followed by four suggested answers or completions. Select **one answer** that is best in each case.

 KNOWLEDGE LEVEL = 1

1. Illicit drugs include:
   A. beer and wine
   B. opiates, cocaine, and amphetamines
   C. alcohol and cigarettes for teens
   D. all of the above

 KNOWLEDGE LEVEL = 1

2. The individuals who are most likely to use illicit drugs are:
   A. 10- to 13-year-olds
   B. 13- to 18-year-olds
   C. 18- to 25-year-olds
   D. none of the above

 KNOWLEDGE LEVEL = 1

3. Indicate the ages of individuals who are most likely to use tobacco and alcohol, rather than illicit drugs.
   A. 10- to 13-year-olds
   B. 13- to 18-year-olds
   C. 18- to 25-year-olds
   D. none of the above

 KNOWLEDGE LEVEL = 1

4. Gateway drugs are defined as:
   A. alcohol, tobacco, and marijuana
   B. cocaine and opiates
   C. amphetamines
   D. all of the above

 KNOWLEDGE LEVEL = 1

5. The leading cause(s) of death among people aged 15–24 years is/are:
   A. violence
   B. accidents
   C. suicides and homicides
   D. all of the above

 KNOWLEDGE LEVEL = 1

6. Among pregnant women, the prevalence of illicit drug use is undefined. However, it is known that heroin use during pregnancy can have which of the following effects?
   A. wide fluctuations in blood levels
   B. premature labor or spontaneous abortion
   C. drug dependency for the infant
   D. all of the above

 KNOWLEDGE LEVEL = 1

7. Which of the following statements defines toxicology?
   A. type of specimen that contains toxins
   B. scientific study and detection of poisons and how they react in the body
   C. legal term meaning illicit drugs
   D. none of the above

 KNOWLEDGE LEVEL = 1

8. Forensic specimens are best described by which of the following statements?
   A. specimens evaluated for civil or criminal legal cases

B. specimens needed to evaluate liver and kidney function

C. tissue specimens from a biopsy sample

D. none of the above

 KNOWLEDGE LEVEL = 1

9. Which of the following may be forensic specimens in certain circumstances?
   A. saliva and teeth
   B. bones, nails, and hair
   C. venous and arterial blood
   D. all of the above

 KNOWLEDGE LEVEL = 1

10. Which of the following statements best defines the chain-of-custody?
    A. specimen transportation vehicle for clinical laboratories
    B. process for maintaining control of specimens from collection to delivery
    C. parental control process for teenagers who abuse drugs
    D. none of the above

 KNOWLEDGE LEVEL = 1

11. A chain-of-custody form must contain the identification of a subject, the time and date of the sample collection, and:
    A. the name of the individual who obtained the specimen
    B. the signature of the subject or patient
    C. a tamper-evident seal
    D. all of the above

 KNOWLEDGE LEVEL = 1

12. After a specimen reaches its destination, the chain-of-custody process requires that:
    A. an armed guard be on the premises during testing phases

B. every individual who handles the specimen sign and complete the chain-of-custody form

C. the specimen is never opened to violate the tamper-evident seal

D. none of the above

 KNOWLEDGE LEVEL = 1

13. The listed acronyms indicate a federal agency and a document that is important to drug testing for federal employees. Identify the correct names for the following: DOT and CCF.
    A. Department of Toxicology and the Center for Criminal Forensics
    B. Department of Transportation and the Center for Custody Forms
    C. Department of Transportation and the Custody and Control Form
    D. Division of Testing and the Custody and Control Form

 KNOWLEDGE LEVEL = 1

14. Professional sports associations such as the National Basketball Association (NBA) and the National Football League (NFL) are among the organizations that have adopted drug-screening programs for their employees. Which of the following statements is accurate in relation to drug-testing employees in these organizations?
    A. Screening is often done without prior notice to the employee.
    B. Procedures for collection and testing are well defined.
    C. Employees being tested must initial the specimen label or seal it.
    D. all of the above

KNOWLEDGE LEVEL = 1

15. According to federal guidelines, collection sites for drug testing can be:
    A. permanent or temporary facilities
    B. in a private home
    C. on a baseball or football field or in a public park
    D. all of the above

 KNOWLEDGE LEVEL = 1

16. Minimum requirements for specimen collection sites to meet federal guidelines for drug testing include which of the following?
    A. The donor must have privacy while providing a urine specimen.
    B. A source must be available for hand washing.
    C. The health care worker must have a work area and must be able to restrict access to the site during collection.
    D. all of the above

 KNOWLEDGE LEVEL = 1

17. Federal guidelines for security measures at sites where specimens for drug screening are collected involve which of the following?
    A. Bluing agents must be added to the toilet bowl accessed by the donor.
    B. Access to water during the urine collection procedure should be restricted.
    C. Unobserved entrances and exits must be prohibited.
    D. all of the above

 KNOWLEDGE LEVEL = 1

18. After a urine sample has been collected for drug testing and the donor gives it to the

health care worker, what is the first thing the health care worker should do?
    A. Read the specimen temperature after 4 minutes.
    B. Check for adequate volume and for evidence of tampering.
    C. Thank the donor for his or her time and escort the donor out.
    D. Seal the specimen.

 KNOWLEDGE LEVEL = 2

19. In drug testing, why would a urine specimen temperature need to be taken after collection?
    A. To check for fever in the donor
    B. To check for infectious bacteria
    C. To check for evidence of tampering
    D. Because some illicit drugs raise the temperature of urine

 KNOWLEDGE LEVEL = 1

20. Circumstances under which a specimen for drug testing might be rejected include which of the following?
    A. The donor's signature is not present.
    B. The seal is missing or shows evidence of tampering.
    C. The chain-of-custody was not signed
    D. all of the above

 KNOWLEDGE LEVEL = 1

21. Which of the following steps can ruin a laboratory result in collecting blood for alcohol levels?
    A. vein selection on the appropriate arm
    B. cleansing the site with alcohol
    C. labeling the specimen so that it cannot be viewed
    D. none of the above

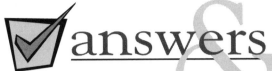

answers & rationales

1.

A. Beer and wine are not defined as illicit drugs.

B. Illicit drugs include opiates, cocaine, amphetamines, and others. (p. 402)

C. Alcohol and cigarette use by teens is not considered illicit, even though such use is harmful and illegal in many cases.

D. "All of the above" is incorrect.

2.

A. Children ages 10–13 are not the most likely to use illicit drugs.

B. Children ages 13–18 are not the most likely to use illicit drugs.

C. Individuals who are most likely to use illicit drugs are in the age category of 18- to 25-year-olds. (p. 402)

D. "None of the above" is incorrect.

3.

A. Children ages 10–13 are not the most likely to use tobacco and alcohol or illicit drugs.

B. Individuals who are more likely to use tobacco and alcohol, rather than other drugs, are in the age category of 13- to 18-year-olds. (p. 402)

C. Adults ages 18–25 are the most likely to use illicit drugs and perhaps to use tobacco and alcohol as well. However, the use of drugs is associated with alcohol and tobacco use at an earlier age.

D. "None of the above" is incorrect.

4.

A. Gateway drugs are alcohol, tobacco, and marijuana. Adolescents with substance abuse problems tend to begin with alcohol and cigarettes, progress to marijuana, and then move on to using other drugs or combinations of drugs. (p. 402)

B. Cocaine and opiates are illicit drugs and are not usually considered gateway drugs.

C. Amphetamines are illicit drugs and are not usually considered gateway drugs.

D. "All of the above" is incorrect.

5.

A. The leading causes of death among people ages 15–24 years are acts of violence, including accidents, suicides, and homicides.

B. The leading causes of death among people ages 15–24 years are acts of violence, including accidents, suicides, and homicides.

C. The leading causes of death among people ages 15–24 years are acts of violence, including accidents, suicides, and homicides.

D. The leading causes of death among people ages 15–24 years are acts of violence, including accidents, suicides, and homicides. (p. 402)

6.

A. It is known that heroin use during pregnancy can cause wide fluctuations in drug blood levels, premature labor, spontaneous abortion, drug addiction for the infant, and other adverse effects.

B. It is known that heroin use during pregnancy can cause wide fluctuations in drug blood levels, premature labor, spontaneous abortion, drug addiction for the infant, and other adverse effects.

C. It is known that heroin use during pregnancy can cause wide fluctuations in drug blood levels, premature labor, spontaneous abortion, drug addiction for the infant, and other adverse effects.

D. It is known that heroin use during pregnancy can cause wide fluctuations in drug blood levels, premature labor, spontaneous abortion, drug addiction for the infant, and other adverse effects. (p. 402)

7.

A. Toxicology is not a type of specimen that contains toxins.

B. Toxicology is defined as the scientific study of poisons, how they are detected, how they react in the body, and the treatment of the conditions they produce. (p. 402)

C. Toxicology is not a legal term meaning illicit drugs.

D. "None of the above" is incorrect.

8.

A. Forensic specimens are those involved in and evaluated for civil or criminal legal cases. (p. 402)

B. Forensic specimens are not specimens needed to evaluate liver and kidney function in a normal patient.

C. Forensic specimens are not necessarily tissue specimens from a biopsy sample, although they may be in certain circumstances.

D. "None of the above" is incorrect.

9.

A. The following may be forensic specimens in certain circumstances: saliva; teeth; bones; nails; hair; venous, capillary, and arterial blood; clothing; dried blood stains; sperm; sweat; and urine.

B. The following may be forensic specimens in certain circumstances: saliva; teeth; bones; nails; hair; venous, capillary, and arterial blood; clothing, dried blood stains, sperm, sweat, and urine.

C. The following may be forensic specimens in certain circumstances: saliva; teeth; bones; nails; hair; venous, capillary, and arterial blood; clothing; dried blood stains; sperm; sweat; and urine.

D. The following may be forensic specimens in certain circumstances: saliva; teeth; bones; nails; hair; venous, capillary, and arterial blood; clothing; dried blood stains; sperm; sweat; and urine. (p. 403)

10.

A. Chain-of-custody does not refer to a specimen transportation vehicle for clinical laboratories.

B. The chain-of-custody is a process for maintaining control of specimens from the time of sample collection to delivery or final disposition of the specimen. (p. 403)

C. Chain-of-custody does not refer to a parental control process for teenagers who abuse drugs.

D. "None of the above" is incorrect.

11.

A. A chain-of-custody form must contain the identification of a subject, the time and date of the sample collection, the name of the health care worker who obtained and processed the specimen, the signature of the subject or patient, and a tamper-evident seal.

B. A chain-of-custody form must contain the identification of a subject, the time and date of the sample collection, the name of the health care worker who obtained and processed the specimen, the signature of the subject or patient, and a tamper-evident seal.

C. A chain-of-custody form must contain the identification of a subject, the time and date of the sample collection, the name of the health care worker who obtained and processed the specimen, the signature of the subject or patient, and a tamper-evident seal.

D. A chain-of-custody form must contain the identification of a subject, the time and date of the sample collection, the name of the health care worker who obtained and processed the specimen, the signature of the subject or patient, and a tamper-evident seal. (p. 403)

12.

A. An armed guard is not necessary on the premises during testing phases.

B. After a specimen reaches its destination, the chain-of-custody process requires that everyone who handles the specimen or an aliquot of the specimen must sign and complete the chain-of-custody form. (p. 403)

C. The specimen must be opened for testing purposes, so the tamper-evident seal will be broken. This is part of the normal process, however, documentation for the chain-of-custody must be maintained.

D. "None of the above" is incorrect.

13.

A. The acronyms DOT and CCF do not represent Department of Toxicology and the Center for Criminal Forensics.

B. The acronym DOT stands for the Department of Transportation, but CCF does not represent the Center for Custody Forms.

C. The acronyms DOT and CCF stand for Department of Transportation, a federal agency, and the Custody and Control Form, a chain-of-custody document that is important to drug testing for federal employees. Standards have been published by the DOT relating to the testing of specimens, quality assurance and quality control, chain-of-custody, personnel, and how results are reported for federal drug testing programs. (p. 404)

D. The acronym CCF stands for the Custody and Control Form, but DOT does not stand for Division of Testing.

14.

A. Drug testing employees in organizations such as the NBA and the NFL usually involves screening without prior notice to the employee, procedures for collection and testing are well defined, and the employee being tested must initial the specimen label or seal.

B. Drug testing employees in organizations such as the NBA and the NFL usually involves screening without prior notice to the employee, procedures for collection and testing are well defined, and the employee being tested must initial the specimen label or seal.

C. Drug testing employees in organizations such as the NBA and the NFL usually involves screening without prior notice to the employee, procedures for collection and testing are well defined, and the employee being tested must initial the specimen label or seal.

D. Drug testing employees in organizations such as the NBA and the NFL usually involves screening without prior notice to the employee, procedures for collection and testing are well defined, and the employee being tested must initial the specimen label or seal. (p. 404)

15.

A. According to federal guidelines, collection sites for drug testing can be permanent or temporary facilities that have privacy during specimen collection and other requirements for the health care worker. (p. 406)

B. A private home would probably not comply with federal guidelines for drug testing facilities.

C. A baseball or football field or a public park would probably not comply with federal guidelines for drug testing facilities

D. "All of the above" is incorrect.

16.

A. Minimum requirements for specimen collection sites to meet federal guidelines are that the donor must have privacy while providing a urine specimen, a source of water or moist towelettes must be available for hand washing, the health care worker must have a work area, and the health care worker must be able to restrict access during the collection process to avoid the possibility of someone tampering with the donor's specimen.

B. Minimum requirements for specimen collection sites to meet federal guidelines are that the donor must have privacy while providing a urine specimen, a source of water or moist towelettes must be available for hand washing, the health care worker must have a work area, and the health care worker must be able to restrict access during the collection process to avoid the possibility of someone tampering with the donor's specimen.

C. Minimum requirements for specimen collection sites to meet federal guidelines are that the donor must have privacy while providing a urine specimen, a source of water or moist towelettes must be available for hand washing, the health care worker must have a work area, and the health care worker must be able to restrict access during the collection process to avoid the possibility of someone tampering with the donor's specimen.

D. Minimum requirements for specimen collection sites to meet federal guidelines are that the donor must have privacy while providing a urine specimen, a source of water or moist towelettes must be available for hand washing, the health care worker must have a work area, and the health care worker must be able to restrict access during the collection process to avoid the possibility of someone tampering with the donor's specimen. (p. 406)

17.

A. Federal guidelines for security measures at sites where specimens for drug screening are collected involve use of bluing agents in the toilet bowl accessed by the donor (to determine whether or not the donor has diluted the urine specimen with toilet water), restricted access to water during the urine collection procedure, the prohibition of unobserved entrances and exits, and secure handling and storage so that the donor need not carry in large bags or articles that can be used to hide a specimen (to substitute for the real one); only collection supplies should be taken into the collection stall.

B. Federal guidelines for security measures at sites where specimens for drug screening are collected involve use of bluing agents in the toilet bowl accessed by the donor (to determine whether or not the donor has diluted the urine specimen with toilet water), restricted access to water during the urine collection procedure, the prohibition of unobserved entrances and exits, and secure handling and storage so that the donor need not carry in large bags or articles that can be used to hide a specimen (to substitute for the real one); only collection supplies should be taken into the collection stall.

C. Federal guidelines for security measures at sites where specimens for drug screening are collected involve use of bluing agents in the toilet bowl accessed by the donor (to determine whether or not the donor has diluted the urine specimen with toilet water), restricted access to water during the urine collection procedure, the prohibition of unobserved entrances and exits, and secure handling and storage so that the donor need not carry in large bags or articles that can be used to hide a specimen (to substitute for the real one); only collection supplies should be taken into the collection stall.

D. Federal guidelines for security measures at sites where specimens for drug screening are collected involve use of bluing agents in the toilet bowl accessed by the donor (to determine whether or not the donor has diluted the urine specimen with toilet water), restricted access to water during the urine collection procedure, the prohibition of unobserved entrances and exits, and secure handling and storage so that the donor need not carry in large bags or articles that can be used to hide a specimen (to substitute for the real one); only collection supplies should be taken into the collection stall. (p. 406)

18.

A. The specimen temperature should be read within 4 minutes but it is not the first step after sample collection.

B. After a urine sample has been collected for drug testing and the donor gives it to the health care worker, the first thing the health care worker should do is to check for adequate volume and for evidence of tampering. (p. 408)

C. The donor should not be allowed to leave until all checks have been made, the specimen has been sealed, initials have been acquired, and the Custody and Control Form has been completed.

D. The specimen should be sealed in the presence of the donor and after required documentation has been completed. This is not the first step after the donor gives the specimen to the health care worker.

19.

A. Urine temperature does not assess fever in the donor.

B. Urine temperature does not assess the presence or absence of infectious bacteria.

C. In drug testing, a urine specimen temperature is taken after collection to check for evidence of tampering. Donors who worry about detection of drugs in their urine may want to dilute the sample with water or other fluids. Normally, fresh urine has a normal body temperature. If cold water (from the toilet or other source) is added to the urine, it will not be at the correct temperature, and tampering is suspected. If this is the case, the health care worker may request another specimen under direct observation according to federal guidelines. (pp. 408–409)

D. Illicit drug use alone does not raise the temperature of urine.

20.

A. Circumstances under which a specimen for drug testing might be rejected include that the donor's signature is not present and there is no indication that the donor refused, the seal is missing or shows evidence of tampering, the chain-of-custody was not signed by the collector, there is insufficient quantity, there has obviously been tampering with the specimen, there is an identification problem, or there is mismatched documentation.

B. Circumstances under which a specimen for drug testing might be rejected include that the donor's signature is not present and there is no indication that the donor refused, the seal is missing or shows evidence of tampering, the chain-of-custody was not signed by the collector, there is insufficient quantity, there has obviously been tampering with the specimen, there is an identification problem, or there is mismatched documentation.

C. Circumstances under which a specimen for drug testing might be rejected include that the donor's signature is not present and there is no indication that the donor refused, the seal is missing or shows evidence of tampering, the chain-of-custody was not signed by the collector, there is insufficient quantity, there has obviously been tampering with the specimen, there is an identification problem, or there is mismatched documentation.

D. Circumstances under which a specimen for drug testing might be rejected include that the donor's signature is not present and there is no indication that

the donor refused, the seal is missing or shows evidence of tampering, the chain-of-custody was not signed by the collector, there is insufficient quantity, there has obviously been tampering with the specimen, there is an identification problem, or there is mismatched documentation. (p. 410)

21.

A. Vein selection on the appropriate arm will not interfere with the test.

B. Cleansing the site with alcohol can ruin a laboratory result when collecting blood for alcohol levels if the health care worker is not careful. A nonalcoholic disinfectant should be used to cleanse the site to avoid contamination of the specimen with the alcoholic disinfectant. (p. 411)

C. Labeling the specimen so that it cannot be viewed should not normally interfere with the test.

D. "None of the above" is incorrect.

Quality Management and Legal Issues

16 Quality, Competency, and Performance Assessment

chapter objectives

Upon completion of Chapter 16, the learner is responsible for the following:

➤ Describe the importance of quality improvement and total quality management.

➤ Describe the 5 D's in terms of negative patient outcomes.

➤ Identify steps in monitoring and evaluating a specimen collection process.

➤ Distinguish between quality control and quality improvement.

➤ Give examples of improved patient outcomes for phlebotomy services.

DIRECTIONS Each of the questions or incomplete statements below is followed by four suggested answers or completions. Select **one answer** that is best in each case.

 KNOWLEDGE LEVEL = 1

1. Dr. W. Edwards Deming had influence in:
   A. hematology instrumentation
   B. phlebotomy standards
   C. quality improvement methods
   D. communication technology

 KNOWLEDGE LEVEL = 1

2. Dr. Avedis Donabedian developed a framework that included key aspects of health care that must be monitored for quality improvement efforts. This framework includes:
   A. hematology and chemistry instrumentation
   B. phlebotomy and results reporting
   C. structures, processes, and outcomes
   D. written and verbal communication

 KNOWLEDGE LEVEL = 1

3. The PDCA cycle represents which of the following?
   A. strategy for quality improvement to plan, do, check, and act
   B. quality model for performing venipunctures
   C. modified Donabedian model
   D. ten-step process for laboratory testing

 KNOWLEDGE LEVEL = 1

4. "Customer satisfaction" is defined as meeting the needs of:
   A. those who are being served
   B. physicians
   C. the JCAHO
   D. those who pay the bills

 KNOWLEDGE LEVEL = 1

5. "CQI" refers to the improvement of health care structures, processes, outcomes, and client satisfaction. QC procedures monitor:
   A. structural aspects
   B. processes
   C. outcomes
   D. client satisfaction

 KNOWLEDGE LEVEL = 1

6. Cause-and-effect diagrams are used in quality improvement methodologies and are designed to assist in:
   A. making bar charts that show the frequency of problems
   B. identifying interactions between people, methods, equipment, and supplies
   C. stimulating creative ideas
   D. breaking out components into a flowchart

 KNOWLEDGE LEVEL = 1

7. Pareto charts are used in quality improvement methodologies and are designed to assist in:
   A. making bar charts that show the frequency of problems
   B. identifying interactions between people, methods, equipment, and supplies
   C. stimulating creative ideas
   D. breaking out components into a flowchart

KNOWLEDGE LEVEL = 1

8. Flowcharts are used in quality improvement methodologies and are designed to assist in:
   A. making bar charts that show the frequency of problems
   B. identifying interactions between people, methods, equipment, and supplies
   C. stimulating creative ideas
   D. breaking out components into a diagram to understand a process

 KNOWLEDGE LEVEL = 1

9. In a health care setting, the customers are:
   A. patients
   B. nurses and other allied health workers
   C. physicians and medical students
   D. all of the above

 KNOWLEDGE LEVEL = 1

10. Quality improvement efforts for specimen collection frequently involve:
    A. phlebotomist's technique
    B. frequency of hematomas
    C. recollection rates
    D. all of the above

 KNOWLEDGE LEVEL = 1

11. Outcomes assessments for quality improvement include:
    A. nosocomial infection rates
    B. the number of fire extinguishers available
    C. the presence of a pathologist 24 hours per day
    D. all of the above

 KNOWLEDGE LEVEL = 1

12. The 5 D's that indicate poor patient outcomes are:
    A. death, disagreement, disruption, dropping a specimen, and defying protocol
    B. death, disease, disability, discomfort, and dissatisfaction
    C. discarding the needle, dropping the specimen, drying the slides, disagreeing with the patient, and defining protocol
    D. all of the above

 KNOWLEDGE LEVEL = 1

13. To reduce blood collection errors, the health care worker should periodically review:
    A. skin puncture procedures
    B. isolation techniques
    C. microcollection techniques for children
    D. all of the above

 KNOWLEDGE LEVEL = 2

14. Quality performance involves several attributes, including efficacy. Define this term.
    A. the degree to which the care provided is relevant to the patient's clinical needs
    B. the degree to which appropriate care is available to meet the patient's needs
    C. the degree to which care of the patient has been shown to accomplish the desired or projected outcome
    D. the degree to which the risk of an intervention is reduced

KNOWLEDGE LEVEL = 2

15. Quality performance involves several attributes, including safety. Define this term.
    A. the degree to which the care provided is relevant to the patient's clinical needs
    B. the degree to which appropriate care is available to meet the patient's needs
    C. the degree to which care of the patient has been shown to accomplish the desired or projected outcome
    D. the degree to which the risk of an intervention is reduced

 KNOWLEDGE LEVEL = 2

16. Quality performance involves several attributes, including availability. Define this term.
    A. the degree to which the care provided is relevant to the patient's clinical needs
    B. the degree to which appropriate care is available to meet the patient's needs
    C. the degree to which care of the patient has been shown to accomplish the desired or projected outcome
    D. the degree to which the risk of an intervention is reduced

 KNOWLEDGE LEVEL = 2

17. Quality performance involves several attributes, including appropriateness. Define this term.
    A. the degree to which the care provided is relevant to the patient's clinical needs
    B. the degree to which appropriate care is available to meet the patient's needs
    C. the degree to which care of the patient has been shown to accomplish the desired or projected outcome
    D. the degree to which the risk of an intervention is reduced

 KNOWLEDGE LEVEL = 1

18. Westgard suggested a 5 Q framework for total quality management for clinical laboratories. The major aspects of this framework is/are:
    A. quality planning and laboratory practices
    B. quality control of processes and quality assessment
    C. quality improvement when problems occur
    D. all of the above

 KNOWLEDGE LEVEL = 1

19. Which of the following variables in specimen processing practices should be subject to quality control and monitoring?
    A. centrifugation
    B. aliquot preparation
    C. readiness for testing
    D. all of the above

 KNOWLEDGE LEVEL = 1

20. Which of the following are preanalytic processes inside the laboratory that are subject to quality reviews and monitoring?
    A. sample treatment
    B. registration, distribution, and storage
    C. centrifugation and making aliquots
    D. all of the above

 KNOWLEDGE LEVEL = 1

21. In restocking supplies for venipuncture, how should supplies be organized?
    A. Newest supplies should be used first.
    B. Oldest supplies should be used first.
    C. Expired supplies should be used first.
    D. none of the above

KNOWLEDGE LEVEL = 1

22. How long should specimens without anticoagulant be allowed to clot?
    A. 5 minutes
    B. 15 to 20 minutes
    C. 30 minutes
    D. none of the above

 KNOWLEDGE LEVEL = 1

23. What should be done if the laboratory personnel suspect that delivery times for specimens are becoming excessive?
    A. Define allowable time limits, and monitor frequency of timing delays.
    B. Report each incident to the patient's nurse.
    C. Identify who is responsible for each delay.
    D. none of the above

 KNOWLEDGE LEVEL = 1

24. Health care workers who perform phlebotomy procedures are often asked to maintain the quality control and preventive maintenance records on:
    A. IV pumps
    B. thermometers and centrifuges
    C. X-ray machines
    D. none of the above

 KNOWLEDGE LEVEL = 1

25. What instrument is used to check the speed of a centrifuge?
    A. sphygmomanometer
    B. radiograph
    C. tachometer
    D. vacillating vortex

 KNOWLEDGE LEVEL = 1

26. Which of the following defines the g force of a centrifuge?
    A. It is relative centrifugal force.
    B. It determines the true force exerted by the centrifuge.
    C. It should be approximately 1000 for 10 minutes for good cell separation.
    D. all of the above

 KNOWLEDGE LEVEL = 1

27. The best source for information for quality assessment of customer satisfaction would be:
    A. *Phlebotomy Handbook* by D. Garza and K. Becan-McBride
    B. patients and family members
    C. medical records
    D. laboratory employees

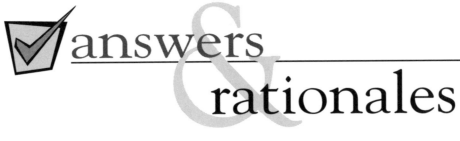

answers & rationales

1.

A. Dr. Deming did not directly influence hematology instrumentation.

B. Dr. Deming did not directly influence phlebotomy standards.

C. Dr. W. Edwards Deming had influence on improving the quality of processes in the manufacturing industry. His focus was on minimizing errors and variations in work processes. His methods have been applied to health care for quality improvement. (p. 426)

D. Dr. Deming did not directly influence communication technology.

2.

A. Dr. Donabedian's framework did not have a direct effect on hematology and chemistry instrumentation.

B. Dr. Donabedian's framework did not have a direct effect on phlebotomy and results reporting.

C. Dr. Avedis Donabedian developed a framework that included key aspects of health care that must be monitored for quality improvement efforts. These key components include structural elements, processes, and outcomes in health care. This framework has guided health care quality improvement measures throughout the recent past. (p. 426)

D. Dr. Donabedian's framework did not have a direct effect on written and verbal communication in health care.

3.

A. The PDCA cycle represents a strategy for quality improvement. It uses a cycle of *planning* the change, *doing* the improvement, *collecting* the data and analyzing the results, *checking* the results to see whether the change improved the situation, and *acting* on what was learned by either rejecting the change, adjusting the change, or adopting the change as a standard part of the process. (p. 427)

B. The PDCA cycle does not represent a quality model for performing venipunctures.

C. The PDCA cycle does not represent a modified Donabedian model.

D. The PDCA cycle does not represent a ten-step process for laboratory testing.

4.

A. Customer satisfaction is defined as meeting the needs of those who are being served. According to this definition, customers can include a variety of groups and individuals within and outside the health care organization. (p. 428)

B. Physicians may also be customers, but they are not the only ones.

C. The JCAHO has a role in regulatory oversight rather than as a customer; however, some might consider JCAHO as a customer who needs to be satisfied with the quality of work.

D. Those who pay the bills (individuals, insurance companies, Medicare, Medicaid, etc.) are also considered customers but are not the only ones.

5.

A. Structural aspects involve physical, personnel, or management or administrative characteristics of an organization.

B. Quality Control (QC) procedures monitor processes. They enable health care workers to adjust analytic processes to meet specific standards. Quality control activities include development of policies and procedures, ensuring that supplies are functional and not outdated, calibrating and maintaining equipment, performing function checks, running QC samples in parallel with patient samples, and participating in proficiency-testing programs. (p. 430)

C. Outcomes refer to what is accomplished for the patient.

D. Client satisfaction involves assessing why customers are happy or dissatisfied with the services provided.

6.

A. Pareto charts are bar charts that show the frequency of problems.

B. Cause-and-effect diagrams are used in quality improvement methodologies and are designed to assist in identifying interactions between people, methods, equipment, and supplies. (pp. 432–433)

C. Brainstorming is a technique to stimulate creative ideas.

D. Flowcharts break out components into a diagram for easier visualization of the process.

7.

A. Pareto charts are used in quality improvement methodologies to show the frequency of problematic events. The Pareto principle suggests that 80% of the trouble comes from 20% of the problems. (pp. 432–433)

B. Cause-and-effect diagrams identify interactions between people, methods, equipment, and supplies.

C. Brainstorming is a technique to stimulate creative ideas.

D. Flowcharts break out components into a diagram for easier visualization of the process.

8.

A. Pareto charts are bar charts that show the frequency of problems.

B. Cause-and-effect diagrams identify interactions between people, methods, equipment, and supplies.

C. Brainstorming is a technique to stimulate creative ideas.

D. Flowcharts are used in quality improvement to break out components into a diagram for easier visualization and understanding of a process. (p. 432)

9.

A. In a health care setting, anyone involved in the health care process both inside and outside of the organization is a potential customer. This includes patients, family members, support groups, all health care workers, those who provide financial support, and vendors of supplies and equipment.

B. In a health care setting, anyone involved in the health care process both inside and outside of the organization is a potential customer. This includes patients, family members, support groups, all health care workers, those who provide financial support, and vendors of supplies and equipment.

C. In a health care setting, anyone involved in the health care process both inside and outside of the organization is a potential customer. This includes patients, family members, support groups, all health care workers, those who provide financial support, and vendors of supplies and equipment.

D. In a health care setting, anyone involved in the health care process both inside and outside of the organization is a potential customer. This includes patients, family members, support groups, all health care workers, those who provide financial support, and vendors of supplies and equipment. (pp. 428–429)

10.

A. Quality improvement efforts for specimen collection frequently involve assessment of the phlebotomist's technique, frequency of hematomas, re-collection rates, and/or multiple sticks on the same patient.

B. Quality improvement efforts for specimen collection frequently involve assessment of the phlebotomist's technique, frequency of hematomas, re-collection rates, and/or multiple sticks on the same patient.

C. Quality improvement efforts for specimen collection frequently involve assessment of the phlebotomist's technique, frequency of hematomas, re-collection rates, and/or multiple sticks on the same patient.

D. Quality improvement efforts for specimen collection frequently involve assessment of the phlebotomist's technique, frequency of hematomas, re-collection rates, and/or multiple sticks on the same patient. (p. 435)

11.

A. Nosocomial infection rates are an example of outcomes that can be assessed for quality improvement purposes. (p. 431)

B. The number of fire extinguishers available would be an assessment of the physical facility. While this is an important element, it has less effect on patient outcomes unless there is a fire in the facility.

C. The presence of a pathologist 24 hours per day is an assessment of the management structure of the facility and also has less effect on the patient outcome unless there is a problem with a laboratory specimen or result.

D. "All of the above" is incorrect.

12.

A. The 5 D's do not refer to death, disagreement, disruption, dropping a specimen, and defying protocol.

B. The 5 D's that indicate poor patient outcomes are death, disease, disability, discomfort, and dissatisfaction. (p. 431)

C. The 5 D's do not refer to discarding the needle, dropping the specimen, drying the slides, defining protocol and disagreeing with the patient.

D. "All of the above" is incorrect.

13.

A. To reduce blood collection errors, the health care worker should periodically review all technical procedures needed in his or her job.

B. To reduce blood collection errors, the health care worker should periodically review all technical procedures needed in his or her job.

C. To reduce blood collection errors, the health care worker should periodically review all technical procedures needed in his or her job.

D. To reduce blood collection errors, the health care worker should periodically review all technical procedures needed in his or her job. (p. 436)

14.

A. Appropriateness is the degree to which the care provided is relevant to the patient's clinical needs. It also relates to doing the right thing for the patient.

B. Availability is the degree to which appropriate care is available to meet the patient's needs.

C. Efficacy is the degree to which the care of the patient has been shown to accomplish the desired or projected outcome. It relates to doing the right thing for the patient. (pp. 427–428)

D. Safety is the degree to which the risk of an intervention is reduced for the patient and the health care worker.

15.

A. Appropriateness is the degree to which the care provided is relevant to the patient's clinical needs. It also relates to doing the right thing for the patient.

B. Availability is the degree to which appropriate care is available to meet the patient's needs.

C. Efficacy is the degree to which care of the patient has been shown to accomplish the desired or projected outcome.

D. Safety is the degree to which the risk of an intervention is reduced for the patient and the health care worker. (pp. 427–428)

16.

A. Appropriateness is the degree to which the care provided is relevant to the patient's clinical needs. It also relates to doing the right thing for the patient.

B. Availability is the degree to which appropriate care is available to meet the patient's needs. (pp. 427–428)

C. Efficiency is the degree to which care of the patient has been shown to accomplish the desired or projected outcome.

D. Safety is the degree to which the risk of an intervention is reduced for the patient and the health care worker.

17.

A. Appropriateness is the degree to which the care provided is relevant to the patient's clinical needs. It also relates to doing the right thing for the patient. (pp. 427–428)

B. Availability is the degree to which appropriate care is available to meet the patient's needs.

C. Efficacy is the degree to which care of the patient has been shown to accomplish the desired or projected outcome.

D. Safety is the degree to which the risk of an intervention is reduced for the patient and the health care worker.

18.

A. Westgard suggested a 5 Q framework for total quality management for clinical laboratories that included quality planning, quality laboratory practices, quality control of processes, quality assessment, and quality improvement when problems occur.

B. Westgard suggested a 5 Q framework for total quality management for clinical laboratories that included quality planning, quality laboratory practices, quality control of processes, quality assessment, and quality improvement when problems occur.

C. Westgard suggested a 5 Q framework for total quality management for clinical laboratories that included quality planning, quality laboratory practices, quality control of processes, quality assessment, and quality improvement when problems occur.

D. Westgard suggested a 5 Q framework for total quality management for clinical laboratories that included quality planning, quality laboratory practices, quality control of processes, quality assessment, and quality improvement when problems occur. (p. 434)

19.

A. The following specimen processing variables should be subject to quality control and monitoring: readiness for testing, aliquot preparation, and centrifugation.

B. The following specimen processing variables should be subject to quality control and monitoring: readiness for testing, aliquot preparation, and centrifugation.

C. The following specimen processing variables should be subject to quality control and monitoring: readiness for testing, aliquot preparation, and centrifugation.

D. The following specimen processing variables should be subject to quality control and monitoring: readiness for testing, aliquot preparation, and centrifugation. (pp. 436–437)

20.

A. The following are preanalytic processes inside the laboratory that are subject to quality reviews and monitoring: sample treatment; sample registration, distribution, and storage; centrifugation and making aliquots.

B. The following are preanalytic processes inside the laboratory that are subject to quality reviews and monitoring: sample treatment; sample registration, distribution, and storage; centrifugation and making aliquots.

C. The following are preanalytic processes inside the laboratory that are subject to quality reviews and monitoring: sample treatment; sample registration, distribution, and storage; centrifugation and making aliquots.

D. The following are preanalytic processes inside the laboratory that are subject to quality reviews and monitoring: sample treatment; sample registration, distribution, and storage; centrifugation and making aliquots. (pp. 436–437)

21.

A. Newest supplies should be used after older unexpired supplies are used.

B. In restocking supplies for venipuncture, the tubes with a shelf life nearest the current date (the oldest unexpired supplies) should be placed so that they are used first. (p. 437)

C. Expired supplies should not be used at all.

D. "None of the above" is incorrect.

22.

A. Five minutes is not adequate time for clot formation.

B. Fifteen to 20 minutes is not adequate time for clot formation.

C. Specimens without anticoagulant are allowed to clot for 30 minutes so that adequate clot formation may take place. (p. 438)

D. "None of the above" is incorrect.

23.

A. If the laboratory personnel suspect that delivery times for specimens are becoming excessive in many cases, they may define allowable time limits, and begin to monitor the frequency and extent of timing delays. (p. 438)

B. Reporting each incident to the patient's nurse may only aggravate the issue without data to support the accusation.

C. Identifying who is responsible for each delay may curb the problem in the short run; however, gathering data about the timing and frequency of the problem would help to justify changes in procedures to improve the situation.

D. "None of the above" is incorrect.

24.

A. The pharmacy department or personnel usually maintains and monitors IV pumps.

B. Health care workers who perform phlebotomy procedures are often asked to maintain the quality control and preventive maintenance records on thermometers, sphygmomanometers, and centrifuges. (p. 439)

C. The diagnostic radiology department personnel usually maintain X-ray machines.

D. "None of the above" is incorrect.

25.

A. Sphygmomanometers are used to take blood pressure.

B. A radiograph is another term for "X-ray."

C. A tachometer is used to check the speed of a centrifuge. (p. 439)

D. There is no such instrument as a vacillating vortex.

26.

A. The g force of a centrifuge is the relative centrifugal force or true force of the centrifuge and measures the efficiency of the instrument. This measurement should be approximately 1000 for 10 minutes for good cell separation in a blood sample.

B. The g force of a centrifuge is the relative centrifugal force or true force of the centrifuge and measures the efficiency of the instrument. This measurement should be approximately 1000 for 10 minutes for good cell separation in a blood sample.

C. The g force of a centrifuge is the relative centrifugal force or true force of the centrifuge and measures the efficiency of the instrument. This measurement should be approximately 1000 for 10 minutes for good cell separation in a blood sample.

D. The g force of a centrifuge is the relative centrifugal force or true force of the centrifuge and measures the efficiency of the instrument. This measurement should be approximately 1000 for 10 minutes for good cell separation in a blood sample. (p. 439)

27.

A. *Phlebotomy Handbook,* by D. Garza and K. Becan-McBride, is also an excellent source of information for quality assessment ideas for specimen collection services. However, speaking with patients and family members themselves or seeking written measurable information from them would provide specific information about improvement opportunities unique to a facility.

B. The best source for information for quality assessment of customer satisfaction would be patients and family members. (pp. 434–435)

C. Medical records are also useful to acquire information about clinical events and may not reflect the patients' feelings and preferences.

D. Laboratory employees are also valuable sources of information about procedural and technical improvement opportunities; however, they may not reflect all feelings and perceptions of the patients themselves.

17 | Legal and Regulatory Issues

chapter objectives

Upon completion of Chapter 17, the learner is responsible for the following:

➤ Define major legal terms, and explain how they relate to the health care setting.

➤ Define risk, and describe the major elements in a risk management program.

➤ Describe the basic functions of the medical record.

➤ Define informed consent.

➤ Describe how to avoid litigation as it relates to specimen collection in a health care environment.

➤ Describe CLIA '88 in perspective to blood collection and transportation responsibilities.

DIRECTIONS Each of the questions or incomplete statements below is followed by four suggested answers or completions. Select **one answer** that is best in each case.

 KNOWLEDGE LEVEL = 1

1. When a health care provider gives aid at an accident, he or she is usually protected through:
   A. informed consent
   B. implied consent
   C. CPR Law
   D. rightful action consent

 KNOWLEDGE LEVEL = 1

2. Failure to act or perform duties according to standards of the profession is:
   A. battery
   B. negligence
   C. criminal action
   D. slander

 KNOWLEDGE LEVEL = 1

3. Which of the following agencies evaluates the safety, clinical efficacy, and medical efficacy of the equipment and supplies used in blood collections?
   A. FDA
   B. EPA
   C. OSHA
   D. JCAHO

 KNOWLEDGE LEVEL = 1

4. Which of the following agencies maintains national surveillance of health care workers' accidental exposures?
   A. FDA
   B. JCAHO

C. OSHA
D. CDC

 KNOWLEDGE LEVEL = 2

5. In legal cases, "what a reasonably prudent person would do under similar circumstances" refers to:
   A. discovery
   B. standard of care
   C. informed consent
   D. implied consent

 KNOWLEDGE LEVEL = 2

6. If a physician orders laboratory tests for diagnosis and the patient comes to the laboratory with a rolled-up sleeve, he or she is giving:
   A. implied consent
   B. informed consent
   C. rightful action consent
   D. preventive consent

 KNOWLEDGE LEVEL = 3

7. A child who refused to have his blood collected was locked in a room by a health care worker and was forced to have his blood collected. This is an example of:
   A. informed consent
   B. invasion of privacy
   C. assault and battery
   D. a misdemeanor

C. EPA

D. CLIA

KNOWLEDGE LEVEL = 2

8. The standard of care currently used in phlebotomy malpractice legal cases involving health care providers is based on the conduct of the average health care provider in which area?

A. city

B. state

C. national community

D. regional community

KNOWLEDGE LEVEL = 1

9. Which legal concept refers to the voluntary permission by a patient to allow touching, examination, and/or treatment by health care providers?

A. implied consent

B. battery

C. informed consent

D. assault and battery

KNOWLEDGE LEVEL = 2

10. The law enacted in 1992 that regulates the quality and accuracy of laboratory testing (including blood collection) by creating a uniform set of provisions governing all clinical laboratories is referred to as:

A. CLIA '88

B. HCFA

C. FDA

D. EPA

KNOWLEDGE LEVEL = 3

11. Which federal agency states that a laboratory with moderately complex or highly complex testing must have written policies and procedures for specimen collection and labeling?

A. FDA

B. HCFA

KNOWLEDGE LEVEL = 1

12. Before a patient's laboratory test results can legally be released, the patient must:

A. express verbal permission

B. tell his or her physician that it is okay

C. provide written consent

D. provide his or her lawyer's consent

KNOWLEDGE LEVEL = 1

13. The legal term for improper or unskillful care of a patient by a member of the health care team or any professional misconduct, unreasonable lack of skill, or infidelity in professional or judiciary duties is:

A. malpractice

B. misdemeanor

C. litigation

D. liability

KNOWLEDGE LEVEL = 1

14. Which of the following legal branches writes regulations that enforce the laws?

A. administrative branch

B. Judicial branch

C. U.S. Supreme Court

D. executive branch

KNOWLEDGE LEVEL = 1

15. One agency affecting regulations on blood collection is HCFA. The abbreviation stands for:

A. Home Care Financing Administration

B. Health Care Financing Administration

C. Health Care Financial Agency

D. Health Care Funding Agency

KNOWLEDGE LEVEL = 1

16. The avoidance of legal conflicts in blood collection through education and planning is considered:
    A. administrative law
    B. executive law
    C. preventive law
    D. preparatory law

 KNOWLEDGE LEVEL = 2

17. When should incident reports involving accidental HIV exposures be reported?
    A. at the end of the work shift
    B. immediately
    C. after 24 hours
    D. after seeing the employee health physician

 KNOWLEDGE LEVEL = 2

18. The type and use of PPE is overseen by the:
    A. OSHA
    B. FDA
    C. EPA
    D. HCFA

 KNOWLEDGE LEVEL = 2

19. Mrs. Harriott, a phlebotomist who collects blood in Valley View Hospital from 6 A.M. to 12 P.M. during the week recently suffered a needle puncture wound when a HIV-positive psychiatric patient from whom she was collecting blood kicked her. Valley View Hospital must report this accidental exposure incident to the:
    A. FDA
    B. EPA
    C. CDC
    D. OSHA

 KNOWLEDGE LEVEL = 2

20. Examination of witnesses before a trial is referred to as:
    A. discovery
    B. statute of limitations
    C. respondent superior
    D. implied consent

 KNOWLEDGE LEVEL = 2

21. All of the following are ways to avoid malpractice litigation *except:*
    A. regularly participating in continuing education programs
    B. reporting incidents within 48 hours
    C. properly handling all confidential communications without violation
    D. obtaining consent for collection of specimens

 KNOWLEDGE LEVEL = 2

22. A nonmedical reason for using medical records from a patient is to:
    A. allow continuity of the patients' care plan
    B. allow for the health care institution's utilization review
    C. provide documentation of the patients' illness and treatment
    D. document communication between the physician and the health care team

 KNOWLEDGE LEVEL = 1

23. The largest area of litigation regarding health care workers (including phlebotomists) is the:
    A. statute of limitations
    B. implied consent principle
    C. informed consent principle
    D. FDA requirements

KNOWLEDGE LEVEL = 3

24. Which of the following is the best example of setting the standard of care for blood collection?
    A. Texas Association of Clinical Laboratory Sciences
    B. Southwest Regional Phlebotomists' Association
    C. California Clinical Laboratory Association
    D. American Hospital Association

 KNOWLEDGE LEVEL = 1

25. Professional negligence in blood collection is the same as:
    A. malice
    B. malpractice
    C. informed consent
    D. implied consent

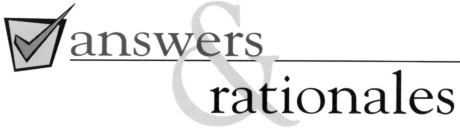

answers & rationales

1.

A. Informed consent is voluntary permission by a patient to allow touching, examination, and/or treatment by health care providers.

B. Implied consent exists when immediate action is required to save a patient's life. (p. 450)

C. Informed consent is voluntary permission by a patient to allow touching, examination, and/or treatment by health care providers.

D. Informed consent is voluntary permission by a patient to allow touching, examination, and/or treatment by health care providers.

2.

A. Battery is the intentional touching of another person without consent; it is also the unlawful beating of another or carrying out of threatened physical harm.

B. Failure to act or perform duties according to standards of the profession is negligence. (p. 445)

C. Criminal actions are legal recourse for acts or offenses against the public welfare.

D. Failure to act or perform duties according to standards of the profession is negligence.

3.

A. The FDA evaluates the safety, clinical efficacy, and medical efficacy of the equipment and supplies used in blood collection. (p. 457)

B. The Environmental Protection Agency (EPA) monitors and enforces environmental requirements for the safe disposal of chemical and biological hazards.

C. The FDA evaluates the safety, clinical efficacy, and medical efficacy of the equipment and supplies used in blood collection.

D. The FDA evaluates the safety, clinical efficacy, and medical efficacy of the equipment and supplies used in blood collection.

4.

A. The Food and Drug Administration (FDA) evaluates the safety, clinical efficacy, and medical efficacy of the equipment and supplies used in blood collection.

B. The Centers for Disease Control and Prevention (CDC) maintain national surveillance of health care workers' accidental exposure.

C. The Centers for Disease Control and Prevention (CDC) maintain national surveillance of health care workers' accidental exposure.

D. The Centers for Disease Control and Prevention (CDC) maintain national surveillance of health care workers' accidental exposure. (p. 448)

5.

A. Discovery is to examine the witnesses before the trial to learn more regarding the nature and substance of each other's case.

B. In legal cases, the standard of care is determined by what a reasonably prudent person would do under similar circumstances. (p. 449)

C. Informed consent is voluntary permission by a patient to allow touching, examination, and/or treatment by health care providers.

D. Implied consent exists when immediate action is required to save a patient's life or to prevent permanent impairment by the patient's health.

6.

A. Implied consent exists when immediate action is required to save a patient's life or to prevent permanent impairment of the patient's health.

236

B. Informed consent is voluntary permission by a patient to allow touching, examination, and/or treatment by health care providers. (p. 449)

C. Informed consent is voluntary permission by a patient to allow touching, examination, and/or treatment by health care providers.

D. Informed consent is voluntary permission by a patient to allow touching, examination, and/or treatment by health care providers.

7.

A. Informed consent is voluntary permission by a patient to allow touching, examination, and/or treatment by health care providers.

B. Invasion of privacy is the physical intrusion upon a person such as the publishing of confidential information.

C. Assault is the unjustifiable attempt to touch another person or threaten to do so in such circumstances as to cause the other to believe it will be carried out. Battery is the intentional touching of another person without consent and the unlawful beating of another or carrying out of the threatened physical harm (i.e., blood collection without consent). (p. 446)

D. A misdemeanor is a general term for all sorts of criminal offenses not serious enough to be classified as felonies.

8.

A. The standard of care currently used in phlebotomy malpractice legal cases and other health care malpractice legal cases is based on the national community as a result of national standards and requirements.

B. The standard of care currently used in phlebotomy malpractice legal cases and other health care malpractice legal cases is based on the national community as a result of national standards and requirements.

C. The standard of care currently used in phlebotomy malpractice legal cases and other health care malpractice legal cases is based on the national community as a result of national standards and requirements. (p. 449)

D. The standard of care currently used in phlebotomy malpractice legal cases and other health care malpractice legal cases is based on the national community as a result of national standards and requirements.

9.

A. Implied consent exists when immediate action is required to save a patient's life or to prevent permanent impairment of the patient's health.

B. Battery is the intentional touching of another person without consent.

C. Informed consent refers to the voluntary permission by a patient to allow touching, examination, and/or treatment by health care providers. (p. 449)

D. Assault is an unjustifiable attempt to touch another person, and battery is the intentional touching of another person without consent.

10.

A. In October 1988, the U.S. Congress passed the Clinical Laboratory Improvement Amendments (CLIA). The law is referred to as CLIA '88 and became effective in 1992 as a means to ensure the quality and accuracy of laboratory testing (including blood collection). (p. 459)

B. The Health Care Financing Administration (HCFA) is the federal agency that administers CLIA regulations.

C. The Food and Drug Administration (FDA) evaluates the safety, clinical efficacy, and medical efficacy of equipment and supplies used in blood collection.

D. The Environmental Protection Agency (EPA) monitors and enforces environmental requirements for the safe disposal of chemical and biological hazards.

11.

A. The Food and Drug Administration (FDA) evaluates the safety, clinical efficacy, and medical efficacy of the equipment and supplies used in blood collection.

B. The Health Care Financing Administration (HCFA) is the federal agency that requires a laboratory with moderately complex or highly complex testing to have written policies and procedures for specimen collection and labeling. (p. 461)

C. The Environmental Protection Agency (EPA) monitors and enforces environmental requirements for the safe disposal of chemical and biological hazards.

D. The Clinical Laboratory Improvement Act (CLIA) is the law over clinical laboratory testing administered by HCFA.

12.

A. Before a patients' laboratory test results can legally be released, the patient must provide written consent.

B. Before a patients' laboratory test results can legally be released, the patient must provide written consent.

C. Before a patients' laboratory test results can legally be released, the patient must provide written consent. (pp. 447–448)

D. Before a patients' laboratory test results can legally be released, the patient must provide written consent.

13.

A. Malpractice is defined as improper or unskillful care of a patient by a member of the health care team or any professional misconduct or unreasonable lack of skill. (p. 448)

B. A misdemeanor is the general term for all sorts of criminal offenses that are not serious enough to be classified as felonies.

C. Litigation is the process of legal action to determine a decision in court.

D. Liability is the obligation to oversee damages.

14.

A. The executive branch writes regulations that enforce the laws.

B. The function of the judicial branch of local, state, and federal government is to resolve disputes in accordance with law.

C. The highest level within the judicial system is the U.S. Supreme Court. The function of the judicial branch is to resolve disputes in accordance with laws.

D. The executive branch writes regulations that enforce the laws. (p. 444)

15.

A. HCFA stands for Health Care Financing Administration.

B. HCFA stands for Health Care Financing Administration. (p. 459)

C. HCFA stands for Health Care Financing Administration.

D. HCFA stands for Health Care Financing Administration.

16.

A. Administrative law is the implementation of statutes and ordinances.

B. The avoidance of legal conflicts in blood collection through education and planning is called preventive law.

C. The avoidance of legal conflicts in blood collection through education and planning is called preventive law. (p. 445)

D. The avoidance of legal conflicts in blood collection through education and planning is called preventive law.

17.

A. An incident report involving accidental HIV exposure should be reported immediately. Actually, any blood collection incident needs to be reported immediately.

B. An incident report involving accidental HIV exposure should be reported immediately. Actually, any blood collection incident needs to be reported immediately. (pp. 452, 456)

C. An incident report involving accidental HIV exposure should be reported immediately. Actually, any blood collection incident needs to be reported immediately.

D. An incident report involving accidental HIV exposure should be reported immediately. Actually, any blood collection incident needs to be reported immediately.

18.

A. The Occupational Safety and Health Administration (OSHA) rule of July 5, 1994, describes the type and use of personal protective equipment (PPE) for health care workers. (p. 457)

B. The Food and Drug Administration (FDA) evaluates the safety, clinical efficacy, and medical efficacy of equipment and supplies used in blood collection but not the rules overseeing personal protective equipment (PPE).

C. The Environmental Protection Agency (EPA) monitors and enforces environmental requirements for the safe disposal of chemical and biological hazards.

D. The Health Care Financing Administration (HCFA) oversees regulations to ensure quality and accuracy of laboratory testing but does not oversee personal protective equipment (PPE) in the laboratory.

19.

A. The Food and Drug Administration (FDA) evaluates the safety, clinical efficacy, and medical efficacy of equipment and supplies in blood collection. It is not engaged in accidental exposure incidents.

B. The Environmental Protection Agency (EPA) monitors and enforces environmental requirements for the safe disposal of chemical and biological hazards. It is not engaged in accidental exposure incidents.

C. Employers are responsible for HIV postexposure follow-up testing. The health care institution must report accidental exposure incidents to the Centers for Disease Control and Prevention (CDC). (p. 448)

D. Employers are responsible for HIV postexposure follow-up testing. The health care institution must report accidental exposure incidents to the Centers for Disease Control and Prevention (CDC).

20.

A. In legal terms, discovery is the right to examine the witness before the trial. (p. 451)

B. In legal terms, discovery is the right to examine the witness before the trial.

C. In legal terms, discovery is the right to examine the witness before the trial.

D. In legal terms, discovery is the right to examine the witness before the trial.

21.

A. To avoid malpractice litigation, it is extremely important to:
- obtain consent for collection of specimens
- regularly participate in continuing education programs
- report incidents immediately and document them
- properly handle all confidential communications without violation.

B. To avoid malpractice litigation, it is extremely important to:
- obtain consent for collection of specimens
- regularly participate in continuing education programs
- report incidents immediately and document them
- properly handle all confidential communications without violation. (p. 452)

C. To avoid malpractice litigation, it is extremely important to:
- obtain consent for collection of specimens
- regularly participate in continuing education programs
- report incidents immediately and document them
- properly handle all confidential communications without violation.

D. To avoid malpractice litigation, it is extremely important to:
- obtain consent for collection of specimens
- regularly participate in continuing education programs
- report incidents immediately and document them
- properly handle all confidential communications without violation.

22.

A. Medical records are sometimes used for nonmedical reasons that are not directly tied to medical services, such as billing, utilization review, and quality improvement within the health care institution.

B. Medical records are sometimes used for nonmedical reasons that are not directly tied to medical services, such as billing, utilization review, and quality improvement within the health care institution. (pp. 452–453)

C. Medical records are sometimes used for nonmedical reasons that are not directly tied to medical services, such as billing, utilization review, and quality improvement within the health care institution.

D. Medical records are sometimes used for nonmedical reasons that are not directly tied to medical services, such as billing, utilization review, and quality improvement within the health care institution.

23.

A. Health care workers are becoming more cognizant of the informed consent principle because this is the largest area of litigation.

B. Health care workers are becoming more cognizant of the informed consent principle because this is the largest area of litigation.

C. Health care workers are becoming more cognizant of the informed consent principle because this is the largest area of litigation. (p. 450)

D. Health care workers are becoming more cognizant of the informed consent principle because this is the largest area of litigation.

24.

A. All health care workers must conform to a specific standard of care to protect patients. In legal cases, the standard of care represents the conduct of the average health care worker in the community. The community has been expanded to the national community and is based on rules and regulations established by national professional organizations.

B. All health care workers must conform to a specific standard of care to protect patients. In legal cases, the standard of care represents the conduct of the average health care worker in the community. The community has been expanded to the national community and is based on rules and regulations established by national professional organizations.

C. All health care workers must conform to a specific standard of care to protect patients. In legal cases, the standard of care represents the conduct of the average health care worker in the community. The community has been expanded to the national community and is based on rules and regulations established by national professional organizations.

D. All health care workers must conform to a specific standard of care to protect patients. In legal cases, the standard of care represents the conduct of the average health care worker in the community. The community has been expanded to the national community and is based on rules and regulations established by national professional organizations. (p. 449)

25.

A. Professional negligence is the improper or unskillful care of a patient by a member of the health care team and is usually referred to as malpractice.

B. Professional negligence is the improper or unskillful care of a patient by a member of the health care team and is usually referred to as malpractice. (p. 446)

C. Professional negligence is the improper or unskillful care of a patient by a member of the health care team and is usually referred to as malpractice.

D. Professional negligence is the improper or unskillful care of a patient by a member of the health care team and is usually referred to as malpractice.

Medical Measurement, Formulas, and Symbols

DIRECTIONS Each of the questions or incomplete statements below is followed by four suggested answers or completions. Select **one answer** that is best in each case.

 KNOWLEDGE LEVEL = 1

1. One inch is equivalent to:
   A. 1 cm
   B. 1 mm
   C. 5 cm
   D. 2.54 cm

 KNOWLEDGE LEVEL = 1

2. One meter is equivalent to:
   A. 36 in.
   B. 39.37 in.
   C. 50 in.
   D. 55.8 in.

 KNOWLEDGE LEVEL = 1

3. One gallon is equivalent to:
   A. 5 L
   B. 4 L
   C. 3.78 L
   D. 1 L

 KNOWLEDGE LEVEL = 1

4. A deciliter (dL) is equivalent to:
   A. 1/2 of a liter
   B. 1/3 of a liter
   C. 1/10 of a liter
   D. 1/100 of a liter

 KNOWLEDGE LEVEL = 1

5. For hematology calculations, the MCV is equivalent to:

   A. hematocrit × 100
   B. hemoglobin × 10
   C. MCH expressed in picograms
   D. hematocrit × 10/RBC count in millions

 KNOWLEDGE LEVEL = 1

6. "Degrees Fahrenheit" refers to:
   A. a unit of temperature
   B. cubic millimeter
   C. a measure of volume
   D. degrees Celsius

 KNOWLEDGE LEVEL = 1

7. The abbreviation QNS refers to:
   A. quality not satisfactory
   B. quantitatively not sound
   C. quantity normally superior
   D. quantity not sufficient

 KNOWLEDGE LEVEL = 1

8. The symbol K refers to:
   A. Kelvin degrees of temperature
   B. kilograms
   C. a unit of volume
   D. kilo-

 KNOWLEDGE LEVEL = 1

9. The symbol < means:
   A. is negative
   B. is greater than
   C. is positive
   D. is less than

KNOWLEDGE LEVEL = 1

10. The symbol L means:
    A. less than
    B. liter
    C. Likert scale
    D. 2.54 cm

KNOWLEDGE LEVEL = 1

11. One cubic centimeter (1 cc) is equivalent to:
    A. 1 kilogram
    B. 1 liter
    C. 1 mL
    D. 1 mCi

KNOWLEDGE LEVEL = 1

12. A candela is a measure of:
    A. energy from heat
    B. luminous or light intensity
    C. time that a candle can burn
    D. distance from a heat source where heat is no longer produced

KNOWLEDGE LEVEL = 1

13. Which of the following symbols represents one cubic millimeter?
    A. mmm
    B. cu mm or mm^3
    C. mL
    D. mM

KNOWLEDGE LEVEL = 1

14. The area of a surface is written in which of the following units?
    A. mass per unit of space
    B. kilogram/liter
    C. cubic meters
    D. square meters or square feet

Military time uses a different method of indicating hours. For Questions 15–19, change the time listed (civilian time) into military time.

KNOWLEDGE LEVEL = 2

15. The military equivalent of 10:16 A.M. is:
    A. 1016
    B. 01000
    C. 0116
    D. 10:16

KNOWLEDGE LEVEL = 2

16. The military equivalent of 3 A.M. is:
    A. 300
    B. 1300
    C. 0300
    D. 2300

KNOWLEDGE LEVEL = 2

17. The military equivalent of 11: 59 P.M. is:
    A. 1159
    B. 2359
    C. 0159
    D. 2159

KNOWLEDGE LEVEL = 2

18. The military equivalent of 1 P.M. is:
    A. 100
    B. 0100
    C. 1100
    D. 1300

KNOWLEDGE LEVEL = 2

19. The military equivalent of 9 P.M. is:
    A. 2100
    B. 2900
    C. 0900
    D. 900

For Questions 20–22, change the time listed (military time) into civilian time to select the correct answer.

 KNOWLEDGE LEVEL = 2

20. The civilian equivalent of 1900 is:
    A. 7:00 A.M.
    B. 7:00 P.M.
    C. 9:00 A.M.
    D. 10:00 P.M.

 KNOWLEDGE LEVEL = 2

21. The civilian equivalent of 0500 is:
    A. 1500
    B. 5 A.M.
    C. 5 P.M.
    D. 5:50

 KNOWLEDGE LEVEL = 2

22. The civilian equivalent of 1448 is:
    A. 2:48 A.M.
    B. 2:48 P.M.
    C. 12:48 P.M.
    D. 4:48 P.M.

 KNOWLEDGE LEVEL = 1

23. Which of the following statements defines RBC distribution width (RDW)?
    A. dispersion of RBC volumes around the mean volume
    B. numerical expression of variation of RBC size
    C. SD of RBC size divided by the MCV
    D. all of the above

 KNOWLEDGE LEVEL = 1

24. One pound is equivalent to how many grams?
    A. 3.78
    B. 453.6
    C. 35
    D. 208

 KNOWLEDGE LEVEL = 1

25. The abbreviation "sp g" refers to which of the following?
    A. specified grams
    B. sufficient glucose
    C. specific glucose value
    D. specific gravity

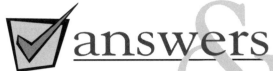

answers & rationales

1.

A. One inch is not equivalent to 1 cm.

B. One inch is not equivalent to 1 mm.

C. One inch is not equivalent to 5 cm.

D. One inch is equivalent to 2.54 cm. (p. 469)

2.

A. One meter is not equivalent to 36 inches.

B. One meter is equivalent to 39.37 inches. (p. 469)

C. One meter is not equivalent to 50 inches.

D. One meter is not equivalent to 55.8 inches.

3.

A. One gallon is not equivalent to 5 L.

B. One gallon is not equivalent to 4 L.

C. One gallon is equivalent to 3.78 L. (p. 469)

D. One gallon is not equivalent to 1 L.

4.

A. 1/2 of a liter

B. 1/3 of a liter

C. A deciliter (dL) is equivalent to 1/10 of a liter. (p. 467)

D. 1/100 of a liter

5.

A. MCV is not equivalent to hematocrit × 100.

B. MCV is not equivalent to hemoglobin × 10.

C. MCV is not equivalent to the MCH expressed in picograms.

D. For hematology calculations, the MCV is equivalent to the hematocrit × 10/RBC count in millions. (p. 472)

6.

A. "Degrees Fahrenheit" refers to a unit of temperature. (p. 473)

B. "Degrees Fahrenheit" does not refer to cubic millimeters.

C. "Degrees Fahrenheit" does not refer to a measure of volume.

D. "Degrees Fahrenheit" does not refer to degrees Celsius.

7.

A. QNS does not refer to "quality not satisfactory."

B. QNS does not refer to "quantitatively not sound."

C. QNS does not refer to "quantity normally superior."

D. The abbreviation QNS refers to "quantity not sufficient." (p. 468)

8.

A. The symbol K refers to Kelvin (a unit of temperature). (p. 467)

B. The symbol K does not refer to kilograms.

C. The symbol K does not refer to a unit of volume.

D. The symbol K does not refer to kilo-.

9.

A. The symbol $<$ does not represent a negative number.

B. The symbol $<$ does not mean "greater than."

C. The symbol $<$ does not represent a positive number.

D. The symbol $<$ means "less than." (p. 468)

10.

A. The symbol L does not mean "less than."

B. The symbol L refers to a liter, a unit of volume. (p. 467)

C. The symbol L does not represent a Likert scale.

D. The symbol L does not represent 2.54 cm.

11.

A. One cubic centimeter (1 cc) is not equivalent to 1 kilogram.

B. One cubic centimeter (1 cc) is not equivalent to 1 liter.

C. One cubic centimeter (1 cc) is equivalent to 1 milliliter (mL). (p. 467)

D. One cubic centimeter (1 cc) is not equivalent to 1 mCi.

12.

A. A candela is not a measure of energy from heat.

B. A candela is a measure of luminous or light intensity. (p. 467)

C. A candela is not a measure of time that a candle can burn.

D. A candela is not a measure of distance from a heat source where heat is no longer produced.

13.

A. One cubic millimeter is not represented by mmm.

B. Cu mm or mm^3 represents one cubic millimeter. (p. 468)

C. One cubic millimeter is not represented by mL.

D. One cubic millimeter is not represented by mM.

14.

A. The area of a surface is not written in mass per unit of space.

B. The area of a surface is not written in kilogram/liter.

C. The area of a surface is not written in cubic meters.

D. The area of a surface is written in square meters or square feet. (p. 471)

For Questions 15–19, civilian time is converted to military time. Military time uses a 24-hour time clock and eliminates the need for "A.M." or "P.M." designations. Time is expressed by up to four numbers; the first set are hours (0–24), and the second set are minutes (0–59). For these questions, only one answer is correct, and all others are erroneous. (p. 472)

15.

A. The military equivalent of 10:16 A.M. is 1016.

B. The military equivalent of 10:16 A.M. is 1016.

C. The military equivalent of 10:16 A.M. is 1016.

D. The military equivalent of 10:16 A.M. is 1016.

16.

A. The military equivalent of 3 A.M. is 0300.

B. The military equivalent of 3 A.M. is 0300.

C. The military equivalent of 3 A.M. is 0300.

D. The military equivalent of 3 A.M. is 0300.

17.

A. The military equivalent of 11:59 P.M. is 2359.

B. The military equivalent of 11:59 P.M. is 2359.

C. The military equivalent of 11:59 P.M. is 2359.

D. The military equivalent of 11:59 P.M. is 2359.

18.

A. The military equivalent of 1 P.M. is 1300.

B. The military equivalent of 1 P.M. is 1300.

C. The military equivalent of 1 P.M. is 1300.

D. The military equivalent of 1 P.M. is 1300.

19.

A. The military equivalent of 9 P.M. is 2100.

B. The military equivalent of 9 P.M. is 2100.

C. The military equivalent of 9 P.M. is 2100.

D. The military equivalent of 9 P.M. is 2100.

For Questions 20–22, military time is converted into civilian time. In military time the first 12 hours are equivalent to the morning, or "A.M.," hours in civilian time. The hours 12–24 represent the evening, or "P.M.," hours in civilian time. For these questions, only one answer is correct and all others are erroneous. (p. 472)

20.

A. The civilian equivalent of 1900 is 7:00 P.M.
B. The civilian equivalent of 1900 is 7:00 P.M.
C. The civilian equivalent of 1900 is 7:00 P.M.
D. The civilian equivalent of 1900 is 7:00 P.M.

21.

A. The civilian equivalent of 0500 is 5:00 A.M.
B. The civilian equivalent of 0500 is 5:00 A.M.
C. The civilian equivalent of 0500 is 5:00 A.M.
D. The civilian equivalent of 0500 is 5:00 A.M.

22.

A. The civilian equivalent of 1448 is 2:48 P.M.
B. The civilian equivalent of 1448 is 2:48 P.M.
C. The civilian equivalent of 1448 is 2:48 P.M.
D. The civilian equivalent of 1448 is 2:48 P.M.

23.

A. RBC distribution width (RDW) is defined as the dispersion of RBC volumes around the mean volume, or a numerical expression of variation of RBC size, or by the calculation below: (p. 472)

$$RDW = \frac{\text{standard deviation (SD) of RBC size}}{MCV}$$

B. RBC distribution width (RDW) is defined as the dispersion of RBC volumes around the mean volume, or a numerical expression of variation of RBC size, or by the calculation below: (p. 472)

$$RDW = \frac{\text{standard deviation (SD) of RBC size}}{MCV}$$

C. RBC distribution width (RDW) is defined as the dispersion of RBC volumes around the mean volume, or a numerical expression of variation of RBC size, or by the calculation below: (p. 472)

$$RDW = \frac{\text{standard deviation (SD) of RBC size}}{MCV}$$

D. RBC distribution width (RDW) is defined as the dispersion of RBC volumes around the mean volume, or a numerical expression of variation of RBC size, or by the calculation below: (p. 472)

$$RDW = \frac{\text{standard deviation (SD) of RBC size}}{MCV}$$

24.

A. One pound is not equivalent to 3.78 grams.
B. One pound is not equivalent to 35 grams.
C. One pound is equivalent to 453.6 grams. (p. 469)
D. One pound is not equivalent to 20.8 grams.

25.

A. The abbreviation "sp g" does not refer to specified grams.
B. The abbreviation "sp g" does not refer to sufficient glucose.
C. The abbreviation "sp g" does not refer to specific glucose value.
D. The abbreviation "sp g" refers to specific gravity. (p. 468)

Index

Page numbers in *italics* denote figures.

Physical medicine department, 17
Physical therapist, 16
Physical therapy department, 18
Physician assistant, 14
Physician review organizations (PROs), 90
Physiology, 31, 32
Pituitary gland, 31
PKU (phenylketonuria), 166–168
Planes of body, 33, 34, 40
Plasma, 52–55, 198
Plastic surgery department, 17
Platelets, 52, 53, 57, 58
Pleural fluid, 205–207
Pneumatic tube systems, 94
Pneumonia, 208
Point-of-care (POC) testing, 196, 199–200
Poison ivy rash, 188
Poisons, 214
Polycythemia, 186
Polymer barrier, 114
Porphyrin, 92
Position of patient
  analytes affected by, 154
  for blood collection, 132, 156, 199
Posterior, 33
Postprandial, 182
Potassium, 118, 122, 155, 197, 198
Potassium hydroxide (KOH) preparations, 39
Potassium oxalate, 115, 117, 118
Povidone-iodine, 114, 135, 147, 179, 186, 189, 190
PPE (personal protective equipment), 13, 14, 238
Preanalytic errors, 96
Preanalytic processes subject to quality review, 229
Pregnancy
  heroin use during, 213
  tests for, 205
Premature infants, 120, 166
  blood volume of, 166, 167
Preventive law, 238
Prilocaine, 168
Primary care, 13, 15, 18
Primary health care workers, 14
PRL (prolactin), 205
Procainamide, 120, 184
Processing errors, 96
Proctology department, 13, 17
Professional sports organizations, drug screening in, 215
Proficiency testing, 89
Prolactin (PRL), 205
PROs (physician review organizations), 90
Protective isolation, 71, 72
Proteus OX 19 assay, 121
Protime (PT), 115, 118, 181
Proximal, 33
Psoriasis, 188
Psychiatry/neurology department, 17
PT (protime), 115, 118, 181
PTT (partial thromboplastin time), 115, 118, 181
Pulmonary arteries, *30, 41*
Pulmonary circuit, *30, 41,* 56
Pulmonary division, 14
Pulmonary veins, *30, 41*
Pulse, 37, 57
Purple-topped blood collection tube, 113, 115, 116, 118–120, 122
Purposes of laboratory analysis, 14

Q

Quality control and improvement, 89, 221–230
Quality control chart, *194,* 198
Quality-control records, 94
Quaternary ammonium compounds, 71

R

Rabies, 70
Radial artery, 55, 180, 187
Radiation exposure, 80, 82
Radiation therapy, 70
Radiograph, 230
Radioisotopes, 11, 15
Radiology department, 11
Radiotherapy section, 18
Rapid plasma reagin (RPR) test, 11, 115, 121
RBCs (red blood cells), 52–54, 57, 58
RDW (red cell distribution width), 247
Reclining position for venipuncture, 132
Rectal diseases, 13, 18
Red blood cells (RBCs), 52–54, 57, 58
Red cell distribution width (RDW), 247
Red-topped blood collection tube, 113, 115, 121, 122
Reference ranges
  for platelets, 57
  for red blood cells, 57–58
Refusal of procedure, 95
Regulatory issues, 231–240
Rehabilitation programs, 18
Rejection of specimens, 138
Renal vein, 54
Renin activity, 116, 122, 198
Reporting laboratory test results, 92, 93
Reproductive system, 31, 34, 38
Requisitions for laboratory tests, 131
Respiration, 36
Respiratory acidosis, 38
Respiratory isolation, 69, 71, 73
Respiratory system, 31, 35, 38
Respiratory tract infections, 69, 71
Restocking supplies, 229
Reverse isolation, 71, 72
Rh phenotyping and genotyping, 15
Rheumatoid factor assay, 11
Rheumatology department, 13
Rocky Mountain spotted fever, 74
Royal blue-topped blood collection tube, 113, 115, 116, 118, 121, 122
RPR (rapid plasma reagin) test, 11, 115, 121
Rubella, 73
Russell Viper Venom (RVV) time, 115, 121

S

S-Monovette, 113, 121
Safe-T-Fill Capillary Blood Collection device, 118
Safety, 76–82, 228–229
Safety-Gard Phlebotomy System, 113
Sagittal plane, 34, 40
Salicylates level, 16
Saline lock, on child, 168
Salivary glands, 37
Salmonella infection, 70, 73
Samplette capillary blood collector, 113, 118
Saphenous veins, 55, 57, 61
Scabies, 70

Scalp vein puncture in infants, 165
Sclerosed veins, 157
Screening newborns for inherited diseases, 166–168
SD (standard deviation), 197–198
Secondary care, 15, 18
Selenium, 115, 122
Seminal fluid, 205
Sensory impairments, 197
Sensory neurons, 36
Sepsis, 147
Serum, 52, 198
  transportation to laboratory, 90
  turbid, 157
Sex determination, 33
Sexually transmitted diseases (STDs), 38
SGOT, 120
SGPT, 120
Sharps container, 80, 120
Shigella infection, 70, 71, 73
Silicon, 114
Simplate R, 188
Sites
  for skin puncture, *142,* 145
  for venipuncture, 53, 132, 136–137, 139
Sitting position for venipuncture, 132
Sizes of vacuum collection tubes, 117
Skeletal system, 33–36
Skin, 11, 15, 34
  blood donation and disorders of, 188
  decontamination before puncture of, 114, 134, 135, 144, 147, 175, 179, 186, 188, 190
  infections of, 70
Skin puncture procedures, 140–148
  for pediatric patients, 166, 167
Skin tests, 206
Sodium, 122, 197, 198
Sodium citrate, 114–119
Sodium fluoride, 114, 115, 119, 121
Sodium heparin, 116, 119
Sodium oxalate, 116
Sodium polyanethosulfonate (SPS), 113, 122, 180–181
Special collection procedures, 169–190
Special handling of specimens, 93
Specialists, 14
Speckled-topped blood collection tubes, 115–117, 119–122
Sperm, 31, 34
Sphygmomanometer, 56, 186, 230
Spina bifida, 166
Spinal cavity, 33
Spinal cord, 36
Spinal fluid, 11, 17, 32, 35, 205
Spleen, 38
Sports organizations, drug screening in, 215
SPS (sodium polyanethosulfonate), 113, 122, 180–181
Sputum analysis, 17
Standard deviation (SD), 197–198
Standard of care, 236, 237, 240
Standard precautions, 72, 74
Staphylococcus aureus infection, 208
"STAT," 135
STDs (sexually transmitted diseases), 38
Steady state, 34
Stem cells, 54